Dr Deepak Ravindran has 20 years of experience in helping people overcome their pain. He is one of the few consultants in the UK with triple certification in musculoskeletal medicine, pain medicine, and lifestyle medicine. Dr Ravindran is a full time NHS consultant in pain medicine and anaesthesia at the Royal Berkshire NHS Foundation Trust in Reading and the lead for the Pain Service.

In 2015, he helped set up the integrated pain and spinal services (IPASS), which provides community pain services for West Berkshire and has been awarded 'Emerging Best Practice' by the British Society for Rheumatology and was shortlisted for a Health Service Journal award. His team won the Grunenthal National Pain Award for General Patient Education in 2017.

Dr Ravindran has been a visiting lecturer at the University of Reading since 2016 and has authored and contributed multiple chapters in many pain management handbooks for healthcare professionals, and patients support groups.

Dr Ravindran is a University Gold Medallist in anaesthesia and pain medicine from one of India's prestigious tertiary super-specialist institutes (JIPMER) and has completed anaesthetic training at Oxford and his pain fellowship at UCL, London.

More recently, he has helped establish the Berkshire Longcovid Integrated Service (BLIS) for managing post COVID syndrome for his local health care system. He lives in Berkshire with his wife and 2 kids.

The
Pain-Free
Mindset

7 steps to taking control
and overcoming
chronic pain

Dr Deepak Ravindran

Vermilion
LONDON

4

Vermilion, an imprint of Ebury Publishing,
20 Vauxhall Bridge Road,
London SW1V 2SA

Vermilion is part of the Penguin Random House group of companies
whose addresses can be found at global.penguinrandomhouse.com

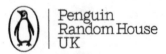

Copyright © Deepak Ravindran 2021
Illustrations © Toby Clarke

Deepak Ravindran has asserted his right to be identified as the author of this
Work in accordance with the Copyright, Designs and Patents Act 1988

First published by Vermilion in 2021

www.penguin.co.uk

A CIP catalogue record for this book is available from the British Library

ISBN 9781785043390

Printed and bound in Great Britain by Clays Ltd, Elcograf S.p.A.

The authorised representative in the EEA is Penguin Random House Ireland,
Morrison Chambers, 32 Nassau Street, Dublin D02 YH68.

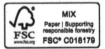

Penguin Random House is committed to a
sustainable future for our business, our readers and
our planet. This book is made from Forest
Stewardship Council® certified paper.

For my teacher, Professor Ravishankar, who embodied wisdom, enthusiasm, passion and curiosity. For inspiring me to deliver value and high-quality care, thank you.

Contents

You do not rise to the level of your goals, you fall to the level of your systems.

James Clear, author of *Atomic Habits*

Introduction

THE FIRST TIME I met Lucy was with her parents in my private clinic. She was very upset and tearful.

'I need you to help me,' said Lucy. 'I've been to so many doctors before and I've just had no clear diagnosis and I need something to get rid of the pain!'

It was heart-wrenching for me to see this young lady sitting there with her equally distraught and worried parents. What had brought their 23-year-old daughter to this situation?

Lucy continued: 'I can't believe it. Up until seven months ago, I was working flat out doing 60-hour weeks at a job I loved and then one day it happened, and from then on everything just went downhill. Nothing has been the same and I just feel so tired. I have pain that is present in every part of my body. Every specialist I've seen gives me a different story and I just want to be put out of this misery.

'It's important that I get this sorted out as soon as possible. I'm at risk of losing my job. I've already taken enough time off work and my boss is just not happy with me. I've got to do better and I am already on notice. This is not worth it. Dr Ravindran – you need to help me; you need to fix this problem.'

Over the course of the next 30 minutes, I realised that Lucy's pain had been gradually building and some opportunities for reducing it early had not been taken. After visiting various specialists, she was not getting any idea of where the problem was, where the pain lay or what could be done to resolve it.

This angst and lack of clarity was what was making it quite difficult for her and her parents. She was at a crisis point and had realised that her job and her life as she knew it, and the quality of life that she used to lead, had all been completely dismantled and taken apart by the pain that was tormenting her all over.

Fast-forward one year and Lucy has just finished her first half-marathon in a very respectable sub-two hours. The work that she did, the support that she had from her parents, and from her larger family and friends, along with the resources that she got from my team, meant that I got the opportunity to witness first-hand something truly transformative.

Lucy was able to achieve all this despite the pain. In fact, she now has a blueprint on how to manage the pain, and look after and pay attention to her body. It was an entirely different Lucy coming to see me in our follow-up appointments or talking on the phone, or even corresponding on social media.

I have now worked with so many patients like Lucy over the last ten years as a NHS consultant practising in a busy district general hospital. I have found a few things that have been instrumental in transforming these patients' attitudes towards their pain and giving them the confidence, ability and belief that they can reach the same position as Lucy: they do not let their pain dictate their life, they have reclaimed their way of living, and have found new purpose and meaning by understanding certain important things about their pain.

In this book, you will understand and learn some very important advances around the treatment of pain, especially developments that have taken place in the last 10–20 years. I'm going to demonstrate that if you can bring these into your life, you could very well achieve the idea of a pain-free existence.

For a large number of you, I am confident that this book will provide the tools to develop a pain-free mindset: an ability to know and understand more about this essential emotion/ sensation of pain that exists within all of us, constantly looking out for us, protecting us, but which sometimes works against us in a misguided attempt to keep us safe.

Lucy, despite her ups and downs, has been able to take this advice and put it to the best use for herself and her life, and it is working with patients like her and seeing the transformation that can come about that prompted me to write this book.

Of course, Lucy's condition and her diagnosis are unique to her, but her problem isn't. She went to many specialists in the NHS, starting with her GP, and then to various allied healthcare professionals, and finally privately to other professionals and clinicians. Lucy had the private insurance to see me quickly, but a lot of patients don't have this and can often wait three or four months before getting an appointment with a pain specialist like me. Additionally, there are not that many experts and teams around who can provide holistic patient support, expectation management and finally patient empowerment, and this lack of knowledge and access to specialists in pain is a problem that has only got worse in the last few years.

Peter's story

Take the case of Peter. He was in his forties and was a baggage handler at a busy airport, and he recollected vividly when his back pain started for him: 'It was a tough day and I didn't have my usual work buddies who would normally help. One was off sick and the other was on annual leave. I was alone on the belt and at one point, when I hoisted a particularly heavy suitcase, I felt something go in the lower part of my back.'

Peter had an initial course of physiotherapy on the NHS. He said, 'I was seen by a physiotherapist the first time. He did an examination and asked me to do a set of exercises and come back in a week's time. When I went the next time, I didn't see the same physiotherapist. Another one came along who looked at the sheet of exercises and had me repeat them. When I went back for the third session, they told me that I could keep doing this and that they would discharge me back to the GP. Nothing more was tested or done.'

When the physiotherapy was not working, Peter was sent for an MRI scan, which showed a small disc bulge in his lower back: 'That frightened the hell out of me. I started getting worried about my ability to walk or lift heavy loads.' This is quite a common story I hear from my patients.

Peter ended up seeing a surgeon privately who felt that the disc bulge would need surgery and that started the first of four surgeries over a period of two-and-a-half years that led to him finally having a spinal fusion that was done about four months ago. The pain continued to get worse after the second surgery, yet, despite this, Peter was operated on a third and fourth time.

Over those four years Peter lost his life. He lost his job and was on long-term sick pay. His relationship with his partner had been affected and they separated. The surgeon had nothing more to offer because they felt that the spinal fusion was solid.

The Problem

The unfortunate reality is that most medical practices and the way a lot of doctors and healthcare professionals in the medical system think still rests on a very flawed assumption that dates from the 1700s: that there has to be a reason for the pain that starts and it only sits with that part of the body that can be removed, blocked, cut or numbed.

This continued persistence of the flawed model – that all pain *always* comes from a structure in the body – is one of the main reasons that chronic pain is poorly understood, poorly managed and poorly treated. If medical professionals are this badly informed, is it any wonder that patients get a raw deal?

Back to basics

At the heart of all this confusion around our knowledge of pain is a 400-year-old philosophy that still guides medical practice up to the present day.[1] René Descartes was a seventeenth-century French scientist and philosopher who was interested in pain, and especially phantom pain. He was the first to propose that pain resided in the brain, which was quite provocative for those times.

Where he went rather awry, given that there were no fancy ways of investigating his claim, was in drawing the pathway of pain as he imagined it. That famous picture suggested that heat, or for that matter any 'painful' sensation, would activate a spot on the skin.

That spot on the skin was attached by a thread all the way to the base of the brain in a structure that we now know as the pineal gland. When that thread pulls on the 'bell' in the brain, it would open up a valve that would allow the 'animal spirits', as it was known at that time, to enter into the muscles, causing a reflex movement of the leg from the source of heat (or pain).

This simplistic assumption that pain was a signal travelling in a thread was a paradigm shift. Descartes' approach (known as the Cartesian model) ensured that the body and the mind could be dealt with separately and gave medical physicians and surgeons the power and ability to open the human body and put it back together again, pursuing treatments that involved cutting, blocking or numbing that thread, and that practice still continues to this day. Prior to this, due to religious beliefs, it was exceedingly difficult to do any surgery or dissection of the human body to understand why people had certain symptoms that made them sick or die. This allowed and spurred the medical progress that we are witnessing up to this day.

Don't get me wrong – the advances in medical science have been indeed revolutionary and we would not have the medications, surgeries or techniques of treatment if it were not for Descartes' reductionistic approach. However, his theory of dualism led to a separation of mental and physical health and, even now, subconsciously, many of us think that mental health is somehow different to physical health. The advances in the last 15–20 years have now shown that dualism is wrong. Understanding how the pathways of emotions are laid out shows that there is a significant link between the mind and the body and each one can affect the other significantly.

Lucy and Peter's stories are very typical presentations that I see in my NHS pain clinic. The first line of defence to deal with any kind of pain is to use over-the-counter tablets. Then, if you have back pain or sciatica-like pain, your GP will often suggest a course of physiotherapy along with some stronger medication. If that doesn't work, you may then be sent for an MRI scan or X-ray to see whether the problem might be a bulged disc or a trapped nerve. If these scans do show some changes, then the journey often involves seeing a surgeon who might or might not suggest further rehabilitation at this time. They may offer an injection or surgery. All of this will be done and, if your symptoms resolve, then that's great.

Unfortunately, one to two out of every five people with this story will not get that benefit and not improve. If you haven't had any acute problem that triggered the pain, like it did for Peter, then it is likely to be muscular. However, your scans may well show some age-related changes, but we won't know nor can we tell for sure whether these changes were sudden or had been happening for some time. At this point, patients are sent to a local pain clinic to see what can be done. This can often happen after a significant period of delay, sometimes as long as two to three years later.[2]

This is a very unsatisfactory way to treat pain, and it needs to change from the outset of the pain, otherwise the chances that it will become persistent start to increase.

The Facts

Chronic pain is now considered to be the biggest pandemic in healthcare today. And if you saw the way we floundered in terms of how we treated patients during the COVID-19 pandemic in 2020, then you can begin to understand how pain also seems to have multiple camps all pushing their line of treatment as the only one that matters.

Pain is a non-communicable disease and causes much productivity loss and economic hardship. In fact, a National Institute for Health and Care Excellence (NICE) report in 2020 estimated that 'arthritis and back pain account for one-third of all claims for disability benefits in the UK' and productivity cost is between £5 billion and £10.7 billion just for back pain.[3] Once you add in the other kinds of pain, such as neck, shoulder or knee pain and migraine headaches, then we are truly talking in numbers that would make the mind boggle.

In my opinion, trying to stick to the 400-year-old habit of wanting to eliminate and get rid of pain by blocking, cutting, removing or incising without *really understanding* the true nature of pain is why we have a healthcare funding crisis in the UK. The prevalence of chronic pain in one recent study has shown that possibly 28 million people in the UK (43 per cent) are struggling with chronic pain.[4] Let's put that into perspective: there are more patients with chronic pain than all of heart disease, diabetes and stroke put together!

You could say that stroke and heart disease are more urgent/important to treat and they can cause death if not treated promptly, but chronic pain is a debilitating condition that you can't see and can't necessarily get rid of without knowing it fully, and it can last a lifetime. A lot of money is spent both by the person and by the system trying to eliminate it using the wrong techniques without even trying to understand it.

Curing pain without understanding its complexity is always going to be a hopeless exercise. Luckily, pain is now much better understood thanks to the works of many excellent researchers in different parts of the world, such as British neuroscientist Irene Tracey and professors like Lorimer Moseley in Australia, who have all contributed to advancing our understanding of pain, and especially chronic pain.

However, the last 15–20 years of stupendous advances have not been made public enough, which means we still subscribe to a flawed theory and continue to keep spending valuable money doing repeated tests, scans, injections and surgeries with very little benefit. We now have the data to say that pain affects almost 20 per cent of the population in most developed and developing countries. This would mean that if we have a population that's close to 8 billion then we are looking at *more than 1.5 billion* with some form of chronic pain not responding to these mainstream medical practices.

Conventional ways don't work

The old way of doing medical practice has got to change. As long as we continue to embrace conventional wisdom, we will always have more chronic pain.

This is something I have learnt the hard way. The good news is that a number of clinicians, including GPs, are now realising the new way forward. There are also many patients who have understood this and many of those outlined in the case studies throughout this book are now active pain advocates who are shining examples of living life meaningfully without necessarily needing medications.

The understanding and support that Lucy had from my team kick-started the changes that she decided to make. She followed a plan and started to notice changes that happened on an incremental basis. She is now empowered to look after herself and understands her body much more than any of the professionals looking after her. She does have her bad days when things are not going exactly right, but she now has the tools and plans to get right back in the saddle.

My Story

I have been looking after patients in pain for 20 years. I have practised pain management in two different continents. I have trained in London and Oxford and I've been a consultant for the last ten years.

Despite doing my pain fellowship and then gaining subsequent qualifications in more specialised interventions and injections for pain management and nerve blocks, I still felt that there were some missing pieces. When I did my diploma in musculoskeletal medicine, I had my epiphany on how much is left to learn and this set me on a journey over the last five years reading and understanding the research. What I found is that pain is not the simple, easy-to-fix problem that I was taught in medical school.

There are often multiple specialists who are interested in managing pain, so rheumatologists, osteopaths, chiropractors, physiotherapists, acupuncturists and, of course, pain specialists and surgeons of multiple specialities are all trying to come at it with their toolbox. In an attempt to achieve that pain freedom, each individual specialist then ends up doing more and more of what doesn't work, and each time you as the patient in pain will still believe that the next treatment will be the final one and will get you pain-free. The reality is very different and will rarely be achieved by just one technique.

Instead, we need to look at pain in a holistic, comprehensive and integrated fashion. If pain management were a game of football, then we need to start by making you a member of the team rather than being the ball that gets kicked about.

I realised that I needed to bring the information in this book not just to my colleagues but also to the most important people – you, the patient. I understand that each form of chronic and persistent pain has its own set of strategies that must be personalised to each patient, but if you can understand what I realised you will have the tools and strategies to conquer your pain and develop a pain-free mindset. My programme works by enhancing your own skills and giving you the confidence that would have disappeared with uncontrolled persistent pain.

Think about how much time has been lost waiting for your next specialist appointment or physiotherapy session. Most people with chronic pain see a healthcare professional for a total of five hours in a year. You need to know what to do for yourself in the remaining 8,755 hours, and that is where this book comes in.

You don't have to wait for the next drug with all its side effects or the next injection/surgery with its chances of failure. With the pain-free mindset, you can take charge of your life and regain control.

How This Book Will Help You

Using the strategies outlined in this book, you will be able to craft your own blueprint to enhance your pain-free mindset, filling your 'backpack' with all the tools you need to help with your pain.

Part 1 gives you the ability and tools to assess where you are in your pain journey. It also outlines what pain really is and helps you to understand the important difference between what I will call 'nociception' and what we know as 'pain'. You'll get the opportunity to use some of the standard questionnaires that I provide for my patients in my NHS practice to help you understand where you are with regard to your pain and nociception, and these will help you take the first steps to developing a pain-free mindset. You'll be able to see for yourself how much you can do to look after your pain and in what circumstances you may need help and support from your GP/specialist.

Part 2 outlines the seven-step MINDSET plan, which my team practises and delivers in the NHS every day: Medications, Interventions, Neuroscience and stress management, Diet/ nutrition, Sleep, Exercise and movement, and finally Therapies of the mind and body. You'll find all the information you need to know about some of the issues and concerns around common pain-relief medications as well as the various interventions, injections and surgeries that are available.

This section will also highlight the critical steps in understanding the power of your nervous system and take you on a whirlwind tour of the influence of diet, nutrition and exercise in overcoming pain. You will see how advanced but complex it has become to understand pain when we see the role of the brain, the intestine and the nervous system in processing various sensations. You will also learn how stress and sleep can impact your pain and that knowing when to sleep and when/what to eat can be as effective in managing your pain as any pill or intervention. I will also cover the hugely important field of therapies that view the mind and body as one whole object, which is now becoming critical in retraining the nervous system and reducing the inflammation in the neuroimmune system, thus reducing stress and pain.

Part 3 will help you to integrate those learnings with your understanding of yourself to create a blueprint for your pain. Once you know more about the pain-free mindset, you will be able to understand what is right for you and where you can get help if it is needed. It's important that you have a clear idea of this so that you can discuss this with your healthcare professional and they can help you with your pain management at the right time with the right technique for the right duration.

Developing a pain-free mindset is the best way forward for long-term pain control. It is not going to be an easy or quick-fix ride, but ultimately this is the most evidence-based, scientifically proven, successful way to take back control of your life, find purpose and meaning, and get back to doing the things that you love.

PART 1

Your Pain Journey

CHAPTER 1

Pain Management Today

ELIZABETH WAS A school teacher who was referred to me by her GP for further management of her neck pain and her constant headaches. She had been given a diagnosis of atypical migraine by her GP and had even seen a neurologist, who had given her a trial of various medications for migraine and headache, but they either weren't effective enough or caused side effects. Her headaches were getting more intense, which meant she had to take time off work.

'I've been informed that there is already a lot of arthritis in my neck and the GP thinks that you can help, but I really don't see how you can make it go away with an injection. I obviously need surgery.

'I've been to so many chiropractors, acupuncturists, osteopaths and a couple of other specialists and they all keep telling me that there's nothing they can do. I'm getting really sick and tired of all of this and this is really not where I want to be. For heaven's sake, I am only 34. This needs to change,' she bristled. 'I think there is something else that's going on, but I don't know what it is and nobody will listen to me.'

This is often the default model when patients go to their GP with chronic pain, not just within the NHS but also in the private sector in the UK and, for that matter, in many other countries around the world. Patients go to their primary care physician and often the first port of call is to a physiotherapist for a brief course of physiotherapy and some exercises. If this works, fantastic. However, if there is very little improvement noted, then patients are referred to a specialist who might be a surgeon or neurologist. Most often, for musculoskeletal pains, which include pains that seem to be coming from any skeletal or muscular part of the body, it is to an orthopaedic physiotherapist or specialist and for any other pain, such as headaches, tummy ache or bladder pain, it is to the relevant specialist surgeon or physician.

Once that specialist has done their share of investigations and looked for a cause to fix, take out or cut but without any success, then the referral is to a pain clinic for further management. And so it was with Elizabeth when she got referred to me.

The problem with this pathway is that a lot of harm is done that is difficult to undo once patients get to this point. In the case of Elizabeth, that harm was as follows:

- The GP clinically made a throwaway remark about a possible disc bulge that started to worry Elizabeth.
- The physiotherapist told her that the pain *should* have resolved after the five sessions of physiotherapy and exercise. Because it hadn't, the physiotherapist believed that there must be something else wrong and had therefore advised further investigation and a referral to a specialist.
- The neurologist told her that it could very well be the disc and ordered a scan. The scan did show the presence of a bulging disc, but it was at another level in her spine and therefore he said that there was no reason for the pain.

- Confused now and still no clearer, Elizabeth became more distressed and her pain started to feel much worse.
- She had another scan done privately and saw a surgeon who advised some steroid injections and an option of surgery by removing the disc if needed or fusing the vertebrae.
- The injection unfortunately did not work and this made the pain worse.

Elizabeth described her neck pain as a constant, intense toothache that never let up. As it got worse, it would go into her head and down to both her shoulders and arms. The terrible thing was that, after all these investigations, Elizabeth had no cause and she still couldn't understand what had happened for her to be in so much pain and why nothing could be done or even seen on the scan.

For her it seemed logical that the disc, even if it was in another place, must be responsible and, while understandably anxious at the prospect of major surgery and more time off work, she felt helpless and had accepted the plan of pursuing surgery as a definite fix.

Many patients wrongly assume that an MRI scan will show the area of pain. That is unfortunately not true at all. An MRI scan shows all the structures – the bones, joints and discs – and all the soft tissues including muscles, ligaments and nerves. However, it only shows structural changes and most of these will occur anyway with age. They are often the wrinkles on the inside! Often those changes do not correlate with the intensity of pain or its location.

What I have found in my clinical practice and with my patients is that it is important to understand the other issues that contribute to the overall pain and use scans and other investigations to see whether there is a clear structural change that is contributing to the pain. In Elizabeth's case it was vital for me to understand who she was as a person and the history of her pain before pre-judging that it all came from one of the structures in her neck.

I sat looking at Elizabeth's scan results and listened to her story, and the distress became evident in her tone as it turned heavy and emotional. The main confusion that she had, and I would have no doubt that many of you would have felt the same in your pain journey, was to have three or four different professionals telling her different variations of the problem with different solutions. Elizabeth had lost time, sleep and quality of life over nearly 18 months without first knowing what the problem was and what she could have done to alleviate her pain.

This all relates to the fundamental understanding that nociception and pain are not the same, and treating one does not treat the other.

The Difference between Nociception and Pain

When you experience an injury and hurt yourself in any part of the body, that perception of hurt activates certain chemicals and channels in your skin and this is called 'nociception'. Nociception occurs in everyone, *but* it is not the same as pain. This is particularly important to understand.

Nociception is what we feel when there is a perception of a harmful signal from a body part. When that information arrives at the brain through a complicated set of nerves, it can be modified at multiple levels by the spinal cord. It is not the simple thread that Descartes thought of (see page 5).

That signal first goes to the spinal cord and then on to multiple areas in the brain, some of which deal with memory, others with emotion, some with logical thinking and others with fear/worry.

This nociception signal pings off these areas of the brain like a ball in a pinball machine and the brain comes up with a final output message. If that message is to seek and get the body to move to safety, it will register in our consciousness as 'pain'. If the outcome from all this pinging is not considered to be dangerous, then there is no pain.

Even though the harm signals (nociception) are happening, the body and brain do not have to express pain. Think about the soldiers who lose their body parts but feel no pain in the heat of the battle. Or the sports player who plays and finishes the game with a fracture!

This is a major shift in understanding pain. Ultimately, pain is to be considered as a signal of danger. That danger is something that the brain has perceived.

The fascinating and challenging part is that this perception of danger can come from sensations within the body (called interoception) or from the external environment (exteroception) without causing any damage to the body. To understand this, we have almost got to move away from that thought we all grew up with: that pain is often an indication of something going wrong in a particular part of the body.

Research over the last 20 years has shown that any harm signal that is generated in a part of the body travels to the nervous system and a common set of chemical signals are produced for a variety of emotions. However, it is finally the spinal cord and the brain that give context to that emotion and *if* they decide that the context is dangerous to the survival of the person then they will express it as pain. This will then make the person seek safety.

This safety can be in any number of ways: retreating into the primitive 'cave' or doing something (medications/intervention) to resolve that danger and feeling of anxiety.

Forty years after the first ever definition of pain, the IASP revised their definition in 2020 and stated that pain is: 'an unpleasant sensory and emotional experience associated with, or resembling that associated with, actual or potential tissue damage'.[1]

They sought to simplify this further for the patient and doctor by stating six key points:

1. Pain is always an experience that is personal and unique to that person.
2. Pain and nociception are very different.
3. People understand what pain is based on their life experiences.
4. Pain is subjective and each person's description should be respected.
5. While pain is there to protect, it can also negatively affect a person's quality of life and well-being.
6. Pain can still be expressed or experienced by people who cannot speak i.e. children/the elderly/those suffering with dementia.

Pain is the sum total of all of the experience and sensation that is processed and put out by the brain, whereas nociception is only a small part of that experience and is a sensation that comes from an actual or deliberate injury or change to the structure arriving at the brain. Unfortunately, our entire medical practice and healthcare runs primarily on thinking

PAIN AND NOCICEPTION

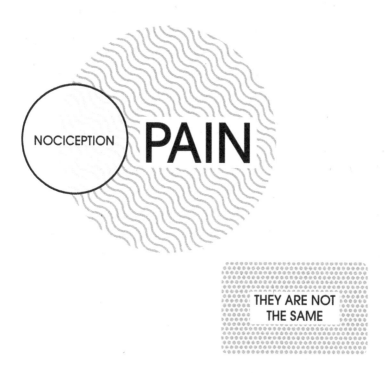

that all of pain is just nociception and that they are one and the same.

In Elizabeth's case, the scan findings and, more importantly, the lack of improvement with a steroid injection meant that there was no inflammatory source in her disc and nerves so nociception was not the reason for her pain. It meant that drugs and injections were not going to be helpful. If she had known how little of her pain was due to nociception then she could have put other measures, such as mind–body therapies, dietary changes and sleep modifications, in place much earlier to ease her pain.

Although we, as healthcare professionals, ask questions and take a good history, we don't often deviate much from our usual set of plans. This applies to all healthcare professionals in general, but, for pain management, if you see a consultant (orthopaedic/pain/surgical), this wrong assumption that nociception always equals pain and that the pain intensity is always proportional to how abnormal a structure looks on a scan means that you'll probably have a discussion around medications and interventions because that is our main expertise.

Nociception responds well to the treatments that we offer in medicine, which include drugs and interventions such as surgery. However, research studies over the last 10–20 years have shown that while medications and interventions are better than some other treatments, they are not great – they don't work for everyone, the risk of harm and side effects is a lot more and, even if they are done very well, 50–70 per cent of patients are left struggling with pain. And if nociception is only a small part of the pain experience and sometimes not there at all, then treating that with drugs and injections is clinically useless.

These are often the only kinds of treatments provided on the NHS, while factors that can make a much bigger difference to the pain – which we'll discuss in Part 2 (pages 41–263) – are not even recognised or reimbursed by insurers or funded on the NHS.

THREE MYTHS I WOULD LIKE TO SHATTER

1. There are pain pathways

Often we are still taught that there are pain pathways. This is a gross oversimplification that allows us to imagine

---

that pain travels in certain pathways that can be interfered with. What we know now is that there are channels and receptors in various parts of the body that pick up harmful signals (chemical or heat) and these 'nociceptive' signals travel within the same nerves to the spinal cord and brain.

2. These signals on arrival to the brain follow certain fixed paths and end at certain structures in the brain and nowhere else

These pathways were thought to be specific and unique and specialised for that emotion, be it pain, mood or anger. We now know that this is not true. In fact, the sensation of nociception is interpreted and processed in multiple parts of the brain. Depending on the context, that signal can be amplified or dampened.

3. Pain always starts from a structure

We now have enough evidence to accept that pain is a signal of danger that could come from within the body or from the external environment. Either of these need not damage the body. We don't have to have a cut, surgery or a fall/injury to feel pain.

When I explain these myths to my patients who are puzzled as to how they can be in so much pain when their X-rays or scans do not show any kind of change, it is a light-bulb moment. I hope it will be the same for you. Now is the time to act and reclaim control.

An Integrated Approach

Tony's story

I first met 48-year-old Tony about three years ago. Being in the building trade, it was much more of a problem when he started to experience chronic low back pain.

It all started as an acute episode about two years prior to the referral when he was on a building site lifting a pallet of heavy bricks. He felt something 'pop' and, as he put it, 'felt something red hot like a poker that started near my left bum cheek and raced down my left leg into the foot.' While that episode took a few weeks to settle down, it then left him with a persistent pain that gradually intensified with time.

This was Tony's fifth follow-up appointment with me in the last eighteen months. I could see that the pain had taken a toll on his life. When he first came, he had had the pain for about nine to ten months and was very keen to 'try anything' to get rid of it and get back to work. When I asked him what he meant by anything, he clarified: 'Any medication, however strong, or, if you feel, surgery.' He obviously very much felt and believed that nociception explained all of his pain.

Now, after 18 months and trials of medication and an injection into the lower back all being ineffective, Tony has started to realise that isn't the quick fix he had hoped for. The weathered, pale face that greeted me this time said, 'Look Dr Ravindran, I have to work otherwise the bills won't get paid. I've got a younger son who is severely autistic and needs care. You need to do something,' he pleaded. 'I don't want to do any more meds. I can't be off with the fairies when I'm on the building site, can I?'

Of course, I could sympathise with that. I've had so many patients telling me that drugs make them feel high and this is a problem with most pain-relief medications. I told him again about all the other non-drug options that could offer similar pain relief and a longer-term sense of control. I had mentioned these at his first appointment but, at that time, his focus was on getting rid of the pain and I don't think he really took it in.

It's so important for clinicians looking after patients in pain to not just stop with their main expertise (be that medications, interventions or physiotherapy), but to actively promote other therapies. Often this is done at the last minute, with perhaps a passing remark before the patient gets up to leave.

We should instead be talking about using a combined approach, rather than focusing most of the consultation on the area of our expertise. Especially with medications or interventions, they should be used as an enabler of further exercise and rehabilitation rather than the only options.

Calming the nervous system and reducing the overall component of the pain is as important as, and I would argue more important than, just trying to reduce the nociception. If there is no active area of nociception, then drugs will not be very effective. This is the reason why patients will often feel that they either don't want to take more drugs, like Tony did, or are afraid to take them because of the side effects.

Another problem that often occurs with drug therapy especially is the habit of doing one thing at a time. In the case of medications, it could be helpful as it avoids the side effects of being on multiple drugs at the same time and not knowing which one is causing the problems. However, it becomes an issue when a patient has an injection and then nothing else. Or when they are asked to stop everything once they have had a course of physio or an injection.

Pain is quite complex and often has multiple reasons. Choosing to employ only one form of therapy first and before trying another that acts on a different pathway defeats the purpose of a multi-pronged way of managing and overcoming the pain.

When we do interventions, there is often no proper rehabilitation plan and sometimes after major surgery all patients are given is a set of exercises and a couple of days of support.

Prem's story

Prem was another classic example of many such patients who come to see me. He was an IT developer who had developed neck pain going to the right shoulder. He was right-handed and developed these symptoms over that last two years. He had some physiotherapy and support through his company insurance, but it did not improve his pain. The GP had prescribed some strong medication (tramadol) but that wasn't effective. Prem also confessed that, because of his work schedule, he wasn't taking it the way it was meant to be taken. Because he didn't have a proper analgesic regime, it was too painful to do the physiotherapy. He went to see one specialist who offered a trial of injections, which gave him an initial improvement, but there wasn't any plan for effective rehabilitation after the injections, so the effect wore off within four weeks. By the time he was in front of me, he had started to run out of ideas.

Prem had done his share of various therapies. However, because he didn't understand the sequence and the reason for doing them, he ended up doing short-term fixes like injections, which neither helped the primary cause nor resolved the issue at hand.

We had a long consultation so we were able to go through his history in a more thorough fashion. Once I showed him where his pain was different from nociception, we put a plan in place to overcome both and bring it all together.

You may think that right now your first desire is to go to the GP or specialist and they will either medicate or inject to take away your pain. Most of modern healthcare and mainstream medicine is incredibly good at treating nociception. *When* it is there. However, when pain has been present for three months or more then nociception is not the target anymore. A long-term condition where there is no nociception but there is pain needs a combined holistic body–mind approach using a variety of resources.

I believe that it is our responsibility as healthcare professionals and organisations to provide as much support and resources as we can in a convenient fashion to make it easy for patients to self-manage. There are many resources available to you if you are confident and know where and how to look. However, if you are in pain it can be difficult to think and remember, and sometimes you need a guide and someone trustworthy to fall back on for advice and reassurance, before you can again be on your way.

This is where this book comes in! *The Pain-Free Mindset* is a seven-step approach that will provide you with all the information and skills you need to manage your chronic pain. It requires a change in mindset to accept the difference between nociception and pain and, no matter which area the pain is coming from, it will show you what your options are if there is a chance that nociception is a big contributor. If you know that there is very little nociception but the pain experience is still high, then you will learn what you can try for yourself and when you need to reach out for help.

Tanya's story

Tanya came to see me with long-standing coccyx (tailbone) pain. Using the principles of dividing nociception and pain, we were able to come up with a set of strategies that addressed the nociception and pain separately. We did a set of simple medication adjustments and a timely injection. At the same time, attention was given to other aspects of posture during sitting and driving, and we optimised her sleep.

Tanya was able to reduce her symptoms by more than 80 per cent within three months and took her first holiday overseas in over ten years. This was a person who had not been able to sit for longer than twenty minutes at a time for more than two years now. She was now able to undertake a short-haul flight to Spain and enjoy her holiday with her partner and kids without having to worry about the pain.

With some simple measures, you can improve so many aspects of your pain and boost your confidence. Doing an assessment of your pain and understanding what your options are is the first step to achieving a pain-free mindset, and this is the focus of the next chapter.

CHAPTER 2

Pain Self-Assessment

TWENTY-FIVE-YEAR-OLD AMY WAS referred to me with back pain. By the time she came to see me, she had tried a variety of medications. She had also had some injections into a couple of joints and nerve blocks with minimal benefit.

In my first session with her, I did a thorough assessment to establish how the pain started, what the history was and what else was happening to her at the time when the symptoms started. If I can understand the entire complexity of a patient's pain story then it gives me various ways in which I can start to make changes; if I can start with that empathy and compassion then it is hugely helpful for the patient. Sometimes I feel this is the most valuable time I can give to my patients.

Within pain management, and probably within most other specialities, often what the patient is expecting from the consultation or treatment is very different to what the healthcare professional can provide, whether that's a drug, an exercise or surgery. Of course, both parties will have their biases and points of view, but inherently, the patient in pain is the more vulnerable party. Danielle Ofri, assistant professor of medicine at New York University School of Medicine, points out this mismatch between the story the patient tells and what the clinician hears. She highlights how patients' stories can be laden with 'layers of emotion, frustration, logistics and desperation, that it was almost as if we were in two different conversations entirely'.[1]

Despite all the high-tech wizardry and gadgets in modern medicine, the single most important thing is the conversation between the clinician and you. The more fancy the surgery, imaging and scans, the more crucial your story, and the latest NICE guidance highlights the importance of this communication and shared decision-making.

When telling her story, Amy realised that this was the first time she had taken a step back and looked at the pain – she could see some connections where there were none before and options to control her pain that were not previously visible to her. When I saw her in a follow-up appointment, she reported that she had noticed a 60 per cent improvement in the intensity of her pain, her sleep was much better and generally she was much happier.

You might be wondering what happened. Amy's improvement was not just due to the medications I had prescribed. They would have helped to an extent, but there were other reasons, with the most critical being that Amy felt more in control; she understood for the first time what the triggers for her pain were and, as long as she took the steps to overcome them, her pain was much improved.

When I have asked some patients what they expect from my appointment before starting, they look at me in a funny way and say, 'You know, make this pain go away.' Though this may be possible in some cases, it is more realistic for you to know what kinds of pain are going to be easily solved and which need a more long-term approach.

There are many types of pain where, after the initial episode, nociception is no longer a major factor. However, the pain can very well become intense, severe and chronic. Some examples of these are:

- headache and neck pain
- back pain
- other osteoarthritis-related joint pain affecting the shoulder, elbow and wrist
- osteoarthritis affecting the hip, knee and ankle joints.
- IBS-related pain
- pelvic pain, either due to previous bladder infection or uterus-related pain
- coccyx (tailbone) pain after posture-related issues or trauma
- nerve damage pain (also called neuropathic pain), either after surgery or accidents, or after conditions like diabetes, hypertension, stroke, Parkinson's, chemotherapy, multiple sclerosis, alcoholism or other toxins/chemical exposures
- others forms of pain like sciatica, sacroiliac pain, tendinitis pain, frozen shoulder, tennis or golfer's elbow
- autoimmune conditions like rheumatoid arthritis, psoriatic arthritis, Crohn's or ankylosing spondylitis
- chronic widespread pain like fibromyalgia, temporomandibular joint pain or interstitial cystitis

Though for many people there may have been some nociception initially (an acute period of chemicals being released), often after a period of time, there will be no further evidence of inflammation, yet the intensity of pain may persist due to other factors, and this will need a different approach than just more medications or interventions.

If you are stuck in a similar kind of cycle in your life right now and you're waiting for your next appointment with your specialist or GP for trials of medications or injections and you feel you've lost control, below are the first tools you need to take back that control and really make a difference to your own pain journey.

You now need to take the time to do a thorough assessment for yourself. You might think that your pain is far too complex and you want somebody else to do this for you, but the questionnaires below only take about 15–20 minutes and will help you to understand the type of pain you are suffering from, the way in which it is affecting your lifestyle and what else can influence it.

The pain questionnaire

Write down your answers to the following questions:

1. It may be difficult to think back to the first time this pain started. However, can you recollect the last time you didn't have any pain at all anywhere? What age were you at that time?

2. What was happening when this pain started? What were you doing? The onset might have been very trivial and you may not even remember it. On the other hand, it could have been after a very traumatic incident, either in a physical or emotional sense.

It is important to know this part because it's the first step to establishing whether there was a component of nociception and how much there was towards the overall pain experience.

3. What have you therefore stopped doing because of the pain? Or, to put it another way, if I could wave a magic wand and completely take away the pain, what you would you want to go back to? This will be a very useful question to you and definitely to your specialist, when you see them.

4. What types of things relieve your pain (e.g. tablets, activities, posture, previous pain treatments, complementary techniques)?

5. What types of things worsen your pain (e.g. tablets, activities, posture, previous pain treatments, emotions, stress)?

6. Over the last three months how many times have you visited or called a medical professional in relation to your pain?

☐ 0–2 ☐ 3–5 ☐ 6–10 ☐ >10

7. Over the past two weeks, has the pain been bad enough to interfere with your day-to-day activities?

☐ Yes ☐ No

8. Over the past two weeks, have you felt worried or low in mood because of this pain?

☐ Yes ☐ No

The body map

Now mark on the drawing opposite the area where you feel pain. Place an 'X' in the place(s) where you feel the pain the most, and indicate by shading where the pain spreads to other parts of your body. Please also describe how the pain feels to you. If it is just one area, that's fine. However, also put down the areas where you have experienced pain in the past. Don't just stop at the joints but also think about whether you had tummy-related pains like irritable bowel syndrome (IBS) or bladder problems.

Chronic pain in itself can be very draining and pain can take away a lot of our belief in ourselves to do things. It can also make us fearful of other activities and pursuits of life, so doing this next exercise will be useful in making you aware whether this is an issue for you.

THE BODY MAP

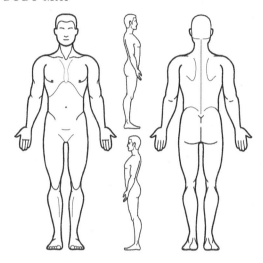

You can find a full-size body map on page 336.

The pain self-efficacy questionnaire (PSEQ)

This questionnaire was created by Professor Michael Nicholas, director of pain education and pain management programmes at the University of Sydney.[2] It is a list of ten questions that will show you how much confidence you have in continuing to do some of your activities while still being in pain. It can include your household chores, socialising, work and your confidence in coping with the pain without medication. It takes less than two minutes to complete and you can check your score on page 39.

Please rate how confident you are that you can do the following things at present, despite the pain. To indicate your answer, circle one of the numbers on the scale under each item, where 0 = not at all confident and 6 = completely confident.

Remember, this questionnaire is not asking whether or not you have been doing these things, but rather how confident you are that you can do them at present, despite the pain.

37

This is very similar to the Patient Activation Measure (PAM®), a widely used measure in primary care.

1. I can enjoy things, despite the pain.

    0   1   2   3   4   5   6

2. I can do most of the household chores (e.g. tidying up, washing dishes, etc.), despite the pain.

    0   1   2   3   4   5   6

3. I can socialise with my friends or family members as often as I used to do, despite the pain.

    0   1   2   3   4   5   6

4. I can cope with my pain in most situations.

    0   1   2   3   4   5   6

5. I can do some form of work, despite the pain ('work' includes housework, paid and unpaid).

    0   1   2   3   4   5   6

6. I can still do many of the things I enjoy doing, such as hobbies or leisure activities, despite the pain.

    0   1   2   3   4   5   6

7. I can cope with my pain without medication.

    0   1   2   3   4   5   6

8. I can still accomplish most of my goals in life, despite the pain.

   0   1   2   3   4   5   6

9. I can live a normal lifestyle, despite the pain.

   0   1   2   3   4   5   6

10. I can gradually become more active, despite the pain.

   0   1   2   3   4   5   6

If you have scored more than 40: You are in the right place to make maximum use of this book and the resources within that are signposted. There is a good chance that you will be able to take back control of your pain.

If you have scored between 20 and 40: You will need to speak to your GP/pain specialist and develop a plan for you to use alongside the learning that you will gain from this book.

If you have scored less than 20: Any gains that you make from treatments, especially medications and injections, may not be long-lasting. You will have to discuss a more personalised and intensive approach with your GP/pain specialist/health coach aided by the material in this book. The aim for you should be to have a holistic plan once the nociception element is reduced.

Amy had a PSEQ score of 42. This helped me understand how confident she felt about her pain and her belief and ability to understand her symptoms.

At our last consultation, she said, 'You're the first person who has been able to be honest with me and say what needs to be done. I needed someone to look at me as a person and help me with an overall plan of what I can do to make myself better. I did not want to be another X-ray that needed to be fixed. I feel much more confident now and know what to do when I get a flare. I have an idea of what is causing it. Most of the time, I know it is due to other factors in my life and I know the things that I can do to reduce and take away the pain sometimes completely.'

You, too, can take control of your pain like Amy. Having completed the exercises above, you now know where you stand in terms of confidence and control and have a good idea of your pain, what it does to you and the other factors that are influencing it. It's time to dive into the core of the pain-free mindset. MINDSET is an acronym covering the most important aspects of pain management:

- **M** is for Medications
- **I** talks about any Interventions
- **N** is the Neuroscience of pain and stress
- **D** reflects the growing role of Diet and the microbiome
- **S** will show you the importance of Sleep for pain
- **E** is the role of physical activity and Exercise
- **T** refers to the Therapies for the mind and body

The information in this book will enable you to discover techniques that work for your pain and may even take it away completely! It will help you to understand why and when drugs and surgeries can work, and what you can do to get the most out of them and the consultations you have with other healthcare professionals. In your journey to overcome your pain, I am confident that knowing these seven steps will form the mindset shift you need to take back control of your life and thrive – pain-free.

PART 2

The Pain-Free MINDSET

CHAPTER 3

Medications

A prescription for a medicine that doesn't work is a prescription for harm: no one wants that.

Dr Cathy Stannard, British pain physician and author

WHEN I FIRST saw Louise's video on her experience with medications, particularly opioids, it brought home to me how much of an adverse impact the medications I prescribe can have on someone's life.[1] She gave a heart-rending account of how the opioids that she thought were life-changing had indeed been that, but in a very different way to what she had hoped for.

It's now been close to four years since she has stopped all drugs and is 'living proof that there really is life after opioids'. However, it has been a long journey that has spanned almost 30 years, and 13 of her important years on ever-increasing doses of strong opioids.

Louise had been given a diagnosis of osteoarthritis and fibromyalgia. Those problems remain, but she is no longer bound to the strong drugs. She is now on the Patient Voice Committee of the British Pain Society as its vice-chair. She has given numerous talks and worked with many organisations to spread the message that it is indeed possible to live well with pain without necessarily needing medication. What changed? How was she different?

I caught up with her and asked her about her experience:

'I have suffered with pain all my life starting from when I was a little girl and I would have aches and pain in my legs and arms, and it would cause me great distress and my mum took me to the doctor. We were told that it was just growing pains and it would go away as I got older, but it never did. It wasn't until my thirties that I got an eventual diagnosis. So in all that time it was quite a bit of a struggle. I've got four grown-up children now and I'm in a different place, but the journey between being the little girl and the grown-up adult was really quite difficult.

'It was really hard for me not knowing what the problem was. People around me started to doubt me because I couldn't say what was going on. It made my working life difficult too. Colleagues weren't very understanding because I couldn't tell them what had been the matter and why I had been off work sick. I worked in a care home with about 40 residents who were elderly, mentally infirm patients and the job was very demanding. I have done it since I was at school and I love the job.'

Initially Louise's GP gave her paracetamol and nonsteroidal anti-inflammatory drugs (NSAIDs) like ibuprofen and naproxen. When they weren't effective, they moved her on to codeine. Finally, she was placed on opioids.

'Initially the opioids meant that my pain diminished greatly and I was able to carry on working and looking after the family and it was almost like a miracle,' she recollected. 'One of my problems was that my back would lock up in the morning. Getting up for work in the morning was a complete nightmare because it took me ages. Opioids made a big difference and it was marvellous – I was able to go back to doing what I was doing before.'

I asked her whether she was given any alternatives to the dosages or the drug itself:

'Not really. Nobody had ever suggested at that point that there might be pain management techniques. I think the first thought back then for me and for the doctors around me was medication.'

When Do Medications Work?

To understand when drugs can work, you need to understand the difference between acute and chronic pain.

Acute pain is a natural response to any form of tissue damage. I introduced you to the difference between nociception and pain on page 20. In acute pain, the amount of nociception is usually quite a large proportion of the total pain experience. This is one reason why acute pain is called nociceptive pain.

When you have an injury like a fracture or surgery where there is damage to the tissue (mechanical, thermal or chemical), then your body, in an attempt to start healing, activates the immune system and creates an inflammatory response, which releases chemicals. These chemicals then sensitise a set of receptors in the area called nociceptors. This sets off a series of signals, some of which travel very fast (causing the sharp pain that you feel) and others that travel slower (responsible for the dull constant ache you have after a tissue injury). These signals reach various parts of the brain, which lets the brain know that there is a danger to which it must react and respond.

As more of the nociceptors get activated, or more chemicals are released in the area, or the duration of the injury is longer,

ACUTE PAIN

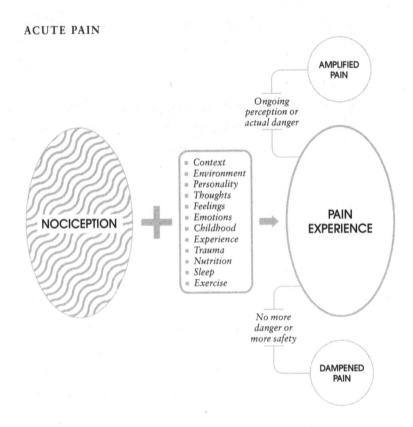

the more severe the pain that is felt. As healing continues, the inflammatory response comes down and the nociceptors don't fire off that often and the pain goes away (in most cases). The brain also understands that it doesn't need to stay on high alert, so it also stands down the alarm system.

Generally, it is assumed that anything could be acute pain for up to a period of three months. If you sustain a tissue injury, like a sprain, or you hurt your knee or ankle, then the general time of healing is between six and ten weeks. So any pain during this period is put down to the inflammation and healing that is going on.

KINDS OF PAIN

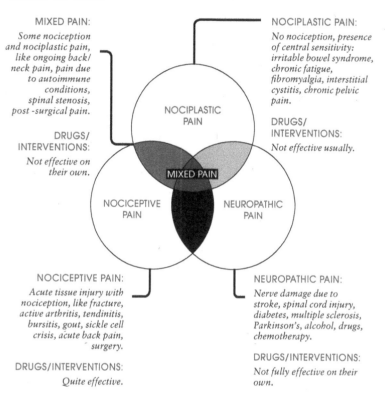

MIXED PAIN:
Some nociception and nociplastic pain, like ongoing back/neck pain, pain due to autoimmune conditions, spinal stenosis, post-surgical pain.

DRUGS/INTERVENTIONS:
Not effective on their own.

NOCIPLASTIC PAIN:
No nociception, presence of central sensitivity: irritable bowel syndrome, chronic fatigue, fibromyalgia, interstitial cystitis, chronic pelvic pain.

DRUGS/INTERVENTIONS:
Not effective usually.

NOCICEPTIVE PAIN:
Acute tissue injury with nociception, like fracture, active arthritis, tendinitis, bursitis, gout, sickle cell crisis, acute back pain, surgery.

DRUGS/INTERVENTIONS:
Quite effective.

NEUROPATHIC PAIN:
Nerve damage due to stroke, spinal cord injury, diabetes, multiple sclerosis, Parkinson's, alcohol, drugs, chemotherapy.

DRUGS/INTERVENTIONS:
Not fully effective on their own.

Very often, in **chronic pain,** there is little nociception. Pain that lasts more than 12 weeks is called chronic or persistent pain. However, chronic pain is not just an extension of the acute pain. It is a totally different entity.

This means that there is often no suggestion of an active inflammation (swelling/redness/temperature raised) that is releasing chemicals and sensitising the nociceptors. There are two categories of this kind of persistent pain: one in which there is proven nerve damage (neuropathic pain) and the other where there is inflammation in the immune system of the brain and spinal cord (nociplastic pain).

In 2019 the World Health Organization (WHO) approved the next version of the 'International statistical classification of diseases and related health problems' (ICD-11) and this will go live in 2022.[2] It marks the first time that chronic pain has been recognised as a separate entity and it will improve patient care by enabling multimodal pain care and allows countries to measure the quality and effectiveness of care. In this model, chronic pain has been divided into broad categories: chronic primary pain and chronic secondary pain:[3]

Chronic primary pain	Chronic widespread pain including fibromyalgia Chronic primary visceral pain (including IBS) Chronic primary musculoskeletal pain Chronic primary headache or orofacial pain (migraine, tension headaches, trigeminal neuralgia) Complex regional pain syndrome
Chronic secondary pain	Chronic cancer-related pain Chronic post-surgical pain Chronic secondary MSK pain (rheumatoid arthritis, osteoarthritis) Chronic secondary visceral pain Chronic neuropathic pain Chronic secondary headache or facial pain

If you have been unfortunate enough to be involved in an injury or have had to go through surgery where some nerves might have been injured then we know that, from the outset, the nerve pain is going to become chronic, meaning that it will last more than three months. This division between acute and chronic pain is often useful in terms of research. In clinical practice, we often find that pain does not correlate with tissue change.

For example, in children who have sustained a fracture and are often put into a cast, pain is usually never a problem after the first few days. We know that healing and inflammation is still going on for a few weeks. However, they don't often complain of pain. Scientists now think that this is due to the fact that the brain doesn't need to feel under threat or danger so it does not need to manifest pain because the fracture site is well protected and supported. It means that the nociceptive signals may still keep reaching the brain as healing and inflammation are ongoing, but the brain is able to realise that it does not need to react to them due to the feeling of safety.

In acute pain, there are nociceptive signals that reach the brain. Then there is the response of the brain to the incoming signals and how it processes them. When there are a lot of nociceptive signals then pain medications can effectively dampen them and reduce the signals, so the brain perceives less pain.

Where do medications work?

First of all, let us start with a fundamental misconception. There are no pain 'killers'. That is a misnomer and it still confuses a lot of my patients when I explicitly tell them that no medications are guaranteed to 'kill' the pain. Instead, they dampen the nociceptive signal and some act on the nervous system and dampen many other signals, and can therefore reduce pain quite effectively.

All the nervous-system-related side effects, like drowsiness, light-headedness, the feeling of being spaced out or sick, are

THE NOCICEPTIVE PATHWAY

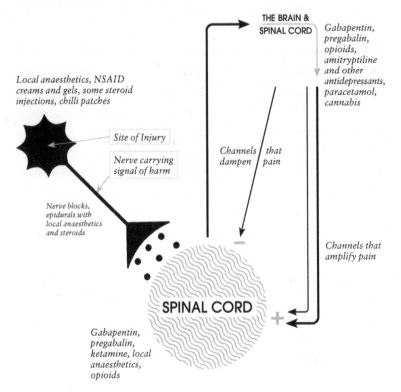

often due to the action of these drugs on various parts of the nervous system. There isn't just one 'pain pathway' (another oversimplification – see page 24) and pain is often sent to multiple parts of the brain. These medications are not selective and end up impacting on other sleep and muscle movement pathways.

However, we do know broadly which part of the nervous system gets affected by each of the drugs and that can often explain what side effects to anticipate. The above pathway shows you at a glance the various parts of the nociceptive pathway and where each of the drugs act.

NOCIPLASTIC PAIN

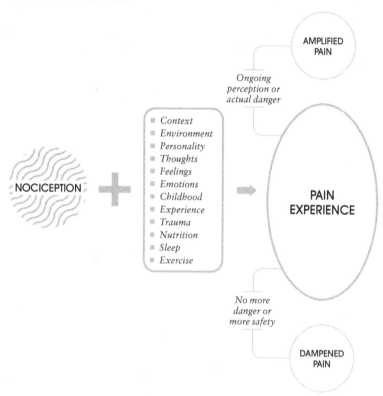

Why Do Medications Not Work?

The kind of constant monitoring of the brain mentioned above can define the entire pain experience. It can amplify the pain experience and make the pain feel worse even though nociception (i.e. the signals from the injury site) hasn't changed. The most important aspect of pain management using drugs is the ability to differentiate between nociception and the whole pain experience.

In most patients with chronic pain, there is very little nociception and a lot of the pain experience is due to changes in the nervous system sensitivity. At a molecular level, it is thought that these may be due to an activation of certain immune cells in the brain/spinal cord called microglia/astrocytes (more on this later – see page 134). This is called nociplastic pain.

A lot of experts consider that the nervous system and the immune system together behave like an oversensitive or incorrectly calibrated alarm system. This makes the nervous system behave very differently and its response to danger and stress signals is vastly different from that of someone who is not in persistent pain.

The faulty alarm system

Think of the nervous system like a burglar alarm system. It is meant to protect us and in acute circumstances, like a forced entry, it is triggered. But what if the internal software or wiring develops a glitch? What if it becomes sensitive to small unnecessary changes?

We recently installed a burglar alarm system in our home after a spate of robberies in the local area. Initially, it was great. It had all the advantages of a modern alarm system; it would alert us to any changes, it had a smartphone app and would notify me when my son came home early or when any door was opened.

Pretty soon, however, it started causing more problems than we had anticipated. We had all been given fobs to activate and deactivate the alarm. When I kept it in my pocket, it would accidentally activate and go off even when there wasn't a burglar. We had one installed in the outhouse and, if the wind got excessive and banged against the doors, the alarm would go off and I would get a notification on my mobile phone app. While I found it initially comforting that it was sensitive, it started to get annoying as it would set off the loud alarm, continuous and deafening, all within the house.

Much like the example above, chronic nociplastic pain can become an unwanted oversensitive burglar alarm and the problem is often within the software. 'Central sensitisation' is the medical term for this bug within the software. If this were an external alarm system, you could switch the whole thing off, but that is not an option with our nervous system. Alternatively, you could put a cloth over the alarm to muffle the noise. Drugs work in the same way – they dampen the alarm in some people, some of the time.

However, that still doesn't solve the problem of the sensor. In an alarm system, you could call the engineer or ask for a replacement sensor. For the human body, we have not as yet found a way to replace the sensor. We are only now realising that the sensor in the software of the brain could be inflamed, but there are no ready drugs available for this at the moment. However, due to the wonderful human nervous system and its plastic adaptive nature, the sensor itself can be retrained to become less sensitive.

My patients often ask me why the sensor gets so sensitive. Professor Lorimer Moseley, a world-famous Australian pain researcher and storyteller, talks about this in an entertaining TED Talk on why things hurt.[4] He gives the example of when he was taking a walk in the woods and felt a scratch on his legs. Shrugging it off, he continued walking until he collapsed soon after. It came to light that what he felt as a scratch was a poisonous snake bite. The nervous system remembered that event and the next time he was walking in the woods and felt another scratch, his system was already primed to take maximum precautions and made him feel the entire experience of pain from the first time around. The difference? The second time around, it really was a twig on the ground.

The brain and nervous system do not take any chances when there is possible danger or threat, so the sensor can become more sensitive if it perceives possible danger or threat, even if it's not there.

The above example can help explain why current pain-relief medications don't work if the issue is of a system under threat. If the danger is perceived or the system thinks that there is danger, drugs cannot stop it nor are they meant to. Drugs can certainly dampen the pain and distract some people, which is what some of the stronger drugs like opioids and muscle relaxants like diazepam do, but their addictive nature causes a separate problem.

Another reason why drugs do not work that effectively is that most pain-relief drugs – at least the strong ones – act mostly on the nervous system. However, we now understand that central sensitisation can become active because of changes in the immune system within the brain or endocrine system, or even diet-related inflammation (because of changes in the microbiome). None of these factors can be helped with our present pain-relief drugs. In short, drugs are unlikely to be effective when it is more a question of the brain having decided that the situation is one of threat and little safety.

In 2019, more than 30 senior researchers looked at all the evidence for medication. They formed part of the development group for the NICE guidance around chronic pain.[5] At the time of writing, they have released a draft of this guidance, which looked at the efficacy of many pain medications and concluded that most drugs, including paracetamol and ibuprofen, aren't effective for these kinds of pains. To say that it caused quite a stir is an understatement!

ARE ALL PAIN MEDICATIONS BAD?

Like any drug, pain medications have their risks and benefits. They are the first line of treatments most often prescribed by specialists and expected by patients. In a rushed ten-minute GP appointment, medications are often the most convenient and quickest way to satisfy both patient and doctor that something has been done. However, what we are discovering is that this is rarely the most appropriate thing to do for patients.

Dr Tim Williams, a GP with an interest in pain, actively suggests that GPs should make longer appointments to discuss persistent pain in more detail before prescribing any medications.[6]

Almost all pain medications have side effects (see page 49). Even the so-called 'simple' drugs like paracetamol can have some problems with prolonged use in some people, so the emphasis is now more on giving short trials of the drugs. Only if they are effective in improving function and/or quality of life are patients then prescribed a particular medication for long-term use.

Common Pain Medications

Drugs given for pain management can be either aimed at reducing the pain or reducing the secondary consequences of being in pain. They can be broadly divided into three categories:

1. Medications primarily for pain: simple analgesics/weak and strong opioids/anti-epileptics and antidepressants/ topical applications.

2. Medications for sleep: some antidepressants and muscle relaxants/zolpidem and zopiclone.
3. Medications for muscle relaxation: diazepam/baclofen.

The table below will give you a good starting point to understand your options regarding pain relief. You may get some of the medications over the counter in the UK, but for most you would need to speak to your GP or a specialist to trial them.

Simple analgesics	Paracetamol and NSAIDs, such as ibuprofen, naproxen, diclofenac.
Weak/moderate-strength opioids	Tramadol, codeine, DF118, dihydrocodeine, hydrocodone.
Strong opioids	Morphine, oxycodone, fentanyl, tapentadol, buprenorphine.
Anti-epileptics	Gabapentin, pregabalin, topiramate, carbamazepine, lamotrigine.
Antidepressants	Amitryptiline, nortryptiline, duloxetine, venlafaxine.
Muscle relaxants	Diazepam, methocarbomol, baclofen.
Topical cream/plasters	Lignocaine 5% plasters, capsaicin 8% patches, capsaicin creams, NSAID creams.
Other new drugs	Botox, low dose naltrexone, cannabinoids, ketamine.

The Faculty of Pain Medicine (FPM) in the UK has a number of high-quality patient information leaflets about common pain medications[7] and several hospitals have also created their own versions of information leaflets about the drugs. The ultimate authority on drug information in the UK is the British National Formulary (BNF).

Simple analgesics, such as paracetamol, can be given first as well as various strengths of codeine, taken individually or in combination. NSAIDs can be tried if there are local muscular components where the pain is worse. Understandably, because of all their risks and problems, opioids (especially strong opioids) are not recommended without specialist advice and support.

The next category of drugs is those that act on various parts of the nervous system, and studies have shown them to be better when it comes to treating central sensitisation. They were initially introduced as antidepressants and anti-epileptic drugs, but now are most often prescribed for pain that is persistent. Especially when we are worried about going down the route of stronger opioids, these drugs are a better alternative. A number of other drugs can be used as 'plasters' for certain conditions.

Herbal treatments

Herbal treatments are very popular, especially in the Eastern cultures of India, China and parts of Africa. The WHO estimates that at least 80 per cent of the world's population uses herbal medicine and often these are recognised as quite effective for the treatment of various medical conditions. Many herbs have an analgesic, anti-inflammatory, antispasmodic and detoxifying or sedating effect.

Some herbs that have been found to be of greater benefit than others include:

Boswellia (frankincense) is an analgesic. It can be used for arthritis, chronic pain from multiple joints, chronic bowel diseases and cancer. It is able to reduce inflammation by stopping leukotrienes, which can cause free radical damage.

Butterbur is a herb found in parts of Europe, Asia and North Africa. It has been used for treating allergies, asthma, headache and muscle spasm. The American Academy of Neurology (AAN) promoted the use of butterbur in their guidelines at a dose of 50–75mg twice daily. When compared to a sugar pill, there is a 48 per cent reduction in headache frequency for those on 75mg of the tablet.[8]

Cat's claw is a vine in the Amazon with anti-inflammatory and antioxidant properties. The bark of this tree is also used in South America to treat a variety of health conditions. Available as capsules in pharmacies and in health food shops, it has been used in both rheumatoid arthritis and osteoarthritis. The side effects are minimal.[9]

Feverfew (a form of chrysanthemum) is often used to prevent migraine headaches. It has been used for a variety of other conditions and gynaecological disorders. In 2012 the AAN listed feverfew as probably effective for migraine prevention.

Ginger is native to the Indian subcontinent and is also grown in Asia, Africa, Latin America and Australia. Ginger has been used for more than 2,500 years as an antimicrobial or antifungal agent.

Green tea has become popular in the last few years. A number of compounds, especially one called epigallocatechin gallate

(EGCG) in green tea, have potent anti-cancer, anti-inflammatory, analgesic, antidiabetic, antibacterial and neuroprotective effects. Numerous studies have shown that EGCG can slow the progression of osteoarthritis.[10]

Curcumin is a herb with anti-inflammatory effects and is native to the Asian subcontinent. It is used in traditional Indian cooking as well as for a variety of medicinal uses. It does have antioxidant, antibacterial, antiviral and anti-inflammatory properties.

How to Take Medications

Assuming that you have some element of nociception or you want to trial pain medications anyway, let's look at what you should look out for and how you should take them.

Firstly, think about small doses of a couple of drugs that influence the signalling pathway (i.e. the signal transmitting fibres). It is important that we use multiple drugs at small doses rather than one drug at a larger dose. Each of these can be started in a stepped manner, meaning that we take a few days with one group before adding in the second type.

I know that may seem unusual, but please hear me out. If you use just one drug at a time and keep thinking that one drug will be enough, then you will find that you need a higher dose over time. This is known as 'tolerance' and you risk running into side effects. However, by using small doses of two or three drugs that act along multiple points of the pathway, you can get the combined benefits of all the drugs while limiting the side effects due to any one drug.

Often, I find that patients are prescribed one drug at a time and, when that doesn't work at a low or a moderate dose, that drug is stopped and another drug is started. This means that many patients cannot take advantage of the combined power of these medications to make a difference to their lives.

The NNT score

The evidence shows and the reality is that most pain medications work only 30 per cent of the time.[11] One remarkably simple and intuitive way to measure the effectiveness of a pain medication in a particular disease condition is with the 'number needed to treat' (NNT) score, which stands for the number of people that one needs to give a certain dose of the medication to (for a certain condition) for one person to get 50 per cent relief.

Generally, it is accepted that a NNT between 2 and 4 is good and worth trialling the drug. A NNT of 1 would be awesome as it would mean that for every one person given the drug, that person would get a benefit of at least 30–50 per cent. A NNT of 7.7 for gabapentin means that up to eight people need to be given the drug for one person to get benefit. Anything higher than that must be carefully weighed up and discussed with you. (Interestingly, if we provided pain education to three people then one person would benefit tremendously simply from education, so the NNT score here would be 3.)

Look at the table on pages 61–2 to identify the NNT for the pain medications that you might be taking or have taken.[12] For example, if you look at ibuprofen, it has an NNT of 2.5, compared to a drug like codeine, which has an NNT of 16. This means that only about three people need to take ibuprofen for one to benefit while sixteen people need to take codeine for one person to benefit.

The high NNT of many drugs and the fact that they are only about 30 per cent effective means that, as clinicians, we need to assess a patient's pain and explore all the options, trialling a few drugs before we get one that works. As one study put it, this means 'asking what works for whom in what circumstance'.[13]

The NNH score

NNH, on the other hand, refers to the 'number needed to harm'. Side effects can occur with any drug and, while many of the side effects are usually well tolerated, some of them can be deal-breakers. For example, I tell patients who are starting on gabapentin and pregabalin that one of the possible side effects is weight gain. That puts a lot of patients off trying the medication.

As you might have guessed, the lower the NNH, the worse the drug. For example, if you have a drug like gabapentin with a NNH of 3.7, it means that for every four people taking the drug, one person is likely to sustain harm (minor side effects like drowsiness and nausea). If you look at drugs like paracetamol or ibuprofen, the NNH is usually in double digits, which is where we generally like them to be.

Drug name	NNT	NNH	Condition
Paracetamol	3–4	12	Acute pain and chronic arthritis
Ibuprofen	2.5	82	Acute pain/arthritis
Naproxen	2.5	135	Acute pain/arthritis
Codeine	16.7	14–20	Acute pain

Tramadol	3.4–4.7 2.4–4.8	8.3	Neuropathic pain Post-surgery pain
Morphine	2.5–4.3	4.2–8.3	Neuropathic pain
Oxycodone	2.5–4.3	4.3–8.3	Neuropathic pain
Gabapentin	7.2–7.7	3.7	Neuropathic pain
Pregabalin	7.7 13–22	3.7	Neuropathic pain/ Fibromyalgia
Amitryptiline and nortryptiline	3.6	6	Neuropathic pain
Venlafaxine and duloxetine	6.4	9.6	Neuropathic pain
Lignocaine patch	4.4	Likely to be quite high	Peripheral nerve pain
Capsaicin patch	10.6	3 (minor side effects)	Peripheral nerve pain
Pain Science Education	3	Likely to be very high	Any persistent pain
Paracetamol and codeine	2.2		Acute pain
Paracetamol and ibuprofen	1.6		Acute pain

Normally, we would prefer medications to have a low NNT and a high NNH – lying to the top right in the graph shown opposite. Stick to the top right when you are having discussions with your GP or specialist regarding your next new medication.

NNH VS NNT

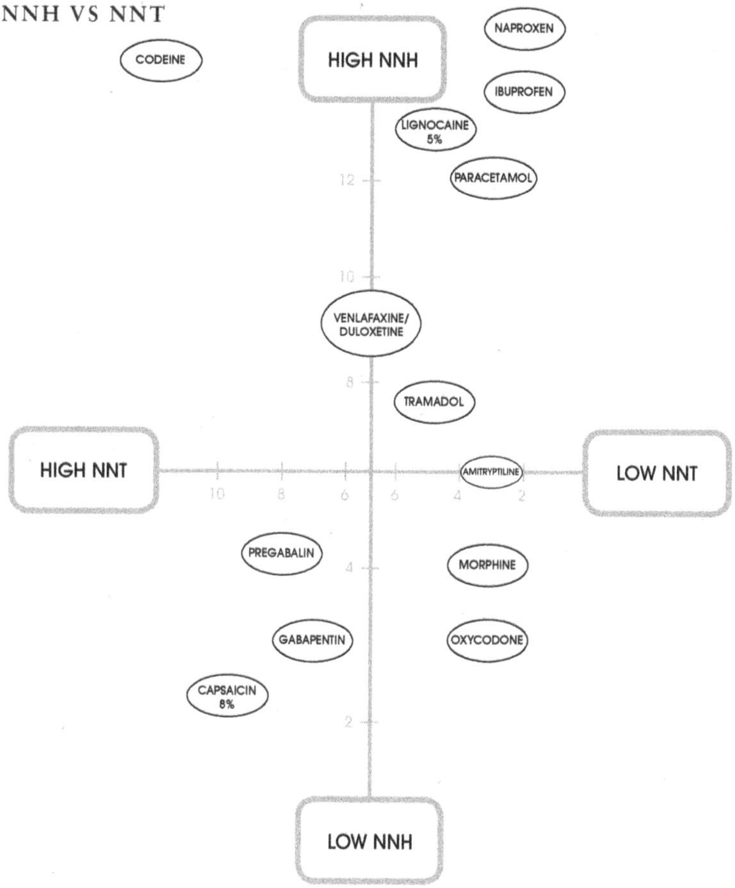
CODEINE
HIGH NNH
NAPROXEN
IBUPROFEN
LIGNOCAINE 5%
PARACETAMOL
12
10
VENLAFAXINE/ DULOXETINE
8
TRAMADOL
HIGH NNT
AMITRYPTILINE
LOW NNT
10
8
6
6
4
2
PREGABALIN
4
MORPHINE
GABAPENTIN
OXYCODONE
CAPSAICIN 8%
2
LOW NNH

Long-Term Side Effects

The problem with harm is becoming very topical and, especially with drugs like opioids, cannabis or gabapentin, the risk of misuse and abuse is often the biggest worry. However, while that puts off a lot of people, the bigger and more common problem is the numerous smaller side effects. They can occur at lower doses, but are more common at higher doses. Sometimes there are some very unusual side effects as well.

Paracetamol	Slightly increased risk of heart problems, bleeding into the digestive system and kidney issues, but quite rare.
NSAIDs	Kidney problems, bleeding into the digestive system, acidity issues, increased risk of strokes/heart attacks/blood clots, bruising, worsening of asthma in some people.
Opioids	Constipation, dependence/addiction, itching, sleep disorders, breathing abnormalities, increased risk of heart failure,[14] heart attacks, excess sensitivity to pain (called opioid-induced hyperalgesia), worsening mood disorders/anger outbursts, increased risk of fractures, decreased level of growth, sex and thyroid hormones and testosterone, lowered immunity, delayed wound healing.
Antidepressants	Sexual problems, inability to reach orgasm, weight gain, worsening mood including suicidal risk, emotionally detached, dependence, withdrawal problems.
Gabapentin and pregabalin	Kidney-related issues, weight gain, dependence and addiction, concentration and memory issues, worsening mood-related issues.

Louise's story

Louise was put on opioids – strong ones like morphine. Initially they worked a treat and she was able to go back to functioning and living well, but soon her pain got worse. Each time the GP increased the dose, she had a temporary period of relief, but then that dose stopped being effective.

'The GP referred me to the pain clinic because he couldn't prescribe anymore. I had never considered and never thought that maybe it was the opiates that were making me so bad until the clinical nurse specialist suggested it. By this time, the pain had got so bad that I was housebound. I didn't make any social plans, couldn't see my grandchildren. My skin sensitivity was through the roof and I couldn't stand people touching me and I didn't want noise.'

This kind of oversensitivity and worsening of pain can be caused by simply increasing the drugs dosage and is seen particularly with opioids. At first, this was thought to be due to underdosing, but we now know that this particular problem occurs with opioids and is called 'opioid hyperalgesia'. It essentially means that the higher the dose (usually above 100mg morphine equivalent total a day), the more chance the drug is making the pain worse. Studies within the brain seem to show that high doses of opioids can cause inflammation and activate various immune cells.[15]

Louise continued: 'Over the next few weeks, every time I went to the nurse in the pain clinic, she would give me something useful to read or a video or website to go away and look at and I wondered if the medication wasn't working at all and maybe she was right; maybe it is the medication. I wondered, if I could get off it quickly, would my life improve?'

At the same time, Louise was starting to have other problems with her skin. She was coming out in boils in many parts of her body and weight gain was becoming an issue. She was having frequent unexplained chest pains for which she needed ambulance call-outs on a couple of occasions. All of this happened on morphine. Once she was switched over to oxycodone, she felt it got much worse. She became much more sensitive throughout her body; she was getting frequent oral infections, painfully sore gums and started to have poor dentition as well. She also writes about the profound impact it had on her sex life and the suppression of her libido due to the opioids.

The final straw that broke the camel's back for Louise were the two emergency admissions to hospital due to severe constipation. The first one started on a Friday with increasing pain and inability to go to the toilet despite taking laxatives. By the Sunday night, the pain had got so intense that an ambulance was called to get her admitted. Louise needed gas and air for the transfer and had to go to the operating theatre to deal with the problem manually.

The feelings of sheer embarrassment and shame were intensified when it happened another time. Louise recollects her second experience: 'The guys in theatre were trying to reassure me that it was okay, I shouldn't be embarrassed. In fact, this was a common thing that they saw with patients on high-dose opioids. I was quite shocked.'

That second episode convinced her that she needed to come off the drugs. She was admitted to the local hospital for an opioid step-down plan. She was understandably worried about withdrawal, but she had great support from her team.

'The withdrawal started to kick in, but the pain wasn't any worse and he (the doctor) reduced it by half the next day and again there was no increase in pain. I had withdrawal symptoms which were extremely odd – I would be crying one minute uncontrollably and remember feeling panic-stricken a few times – but I wasn't in any more pain. In fact, by the third day it had started to improve.'

Louise was 25 stone at the time of her hospital admission and over time has lost 8.5 stone by a combination of coming off the drugs, moving more and watching her nutrition. It has also helped her osteoarthritis and now she can walk without any walking aids. Apart from the occasional paracetamol for her knees, she has not taken any other pain medications for the last three years.

Now you may think that Louise is an outlier. However, I can assure you that I have one or two patients every week in my clinics who are not taking any drugs and manage their pain in completely different ways. The common theme that I have found in all these patients, including Louise, is that they often have a form of movement-based alternative to help with their pain management. They all also practise some form of mindfulness-based skill to enhance the ability of the brain to dampen the central sensitisation. Since there is no or minimal nociception, the pain experience can be managed, and sometimes very effectively reduced, with just the power of the mind. The stress reduction that comes from these techniques calms the brain's immune cells, thus bringing balance. This is very possible and I will talk in more detail about movement and mindfulness in Chapters 8 and 9.

Addiction

Addiction to pain medications is often the main unspoken worry. Certainly these fears were paramount in the fifties and sixties with morphine, and doctors were generally very cautious. However, pain management for patients was still very poor.

Meanwhile, medicine continued to innovate and make rapid breakthroughs. More challenging and longer surgeries were being done and treatments for cancer were being offered that increased the risk of more patients having long-term pain issues, either due to the cancer or due to the chemotherapy or radiotherapy.

Then in the eighties and nineties, the situation started to change. Hospitals in the US began to be judged as good or bad based on how much pain relief patients had at the time of discharge after treatment/surgery. If a patient at the time of discharge was given a strong opioid then they certainly might become pain-free, thus giving a positive feedback. This became part of a score that reflected how hospitals got paid. This skewed healthcare incentive scheme allowed for more opioids being prescribed in larger quantities to more people.[16]

In parallel, an unfortunate alliance between the well-intentioned efforts of doctors to relieve pain and unethical marketing practices of pharmaceutical companies allowed for the ongoing prescription of these drugs in the community to more and more people without really understanding the person in pain or the reasons for that pain.

Addiction as a long-term brain disease

Addiction and dependence are complicated subjects. For a long time, it was considered a moral responsibility and personal failing if someone got addicted. When it was poorly understood, it was easy to paint the problem as something that could be changed if the addict tried hard enough to stop taking drugs. I suspect even now many healthcare professionals and members of the public harbour such a view. However, as the understanding of the brain has evolved we have come to realise that addiction is a chronic brain disease.

Cocaine has been the poster child for addictive drugs and almost all medical professionals know of the experiments that were conducted on rats in cages in the late sixties and early seventies. These seemed to indicate that rats would

ADDICTION PATHWAY

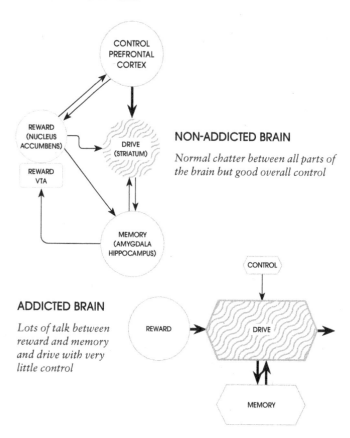

NON-ADDICTED BRAIN

Normal chatter between all parts of the brain but good overall control

ADDICTED BRAIN

Lots of talk between reward and memory and drive with very little control

prefer cocaine-laced water even when other foods were offered to them. This painted a picture of drugs being able to instantly 'hook' a person, even with one exposure. This created a great deal of fear in those times against all opioids including morphine.

The Rat Park experiments of the mid-seventies by Canadian psychologist Bruce Alexander and his team proved very convincingly that when an enriched and supportive environment is available, the rats do not get 'addicted' in the same way as we would expect.[17] In one of the experiments, he exposed rats to 57 days of only morphine-laced water. When he then moved them into Rat Park and they were offered the amenities of the new place, they didn't need the morphine water anymore.

During the Vietnam War in the seventies, there was evidence of widespread cocaine and heroin use amongst the soldiers and it was estimated that up to 15 per cent of the soldiers would be addicted to them permanently. This then prompted a study by Lee Robins, noted psychiatrist and researcher with the US army at that time, and colleagues. In findings that were completely contradictory to existing beliefs at the time, Robins showed that only 5 per cent of the returning veterans got re-addicted on return and only 12 per cent relapsed.[18]

We understand now that the social and economic challenges that many vulnerable patients face and that can maintain addiction are due to a less than satisfactory environment. This point is clearly highlighted by Gabor Maté in his book *In the Realm of Hungry Ghosts: Close encounters with addiction*.[19] Dr Maté is a Canadian general physician and an expert on addictions and served as the resident physician at the Portland Hospital in downtown Vancouver. His harrowing and emotionally charged accounts of the reasons for addiction and trauma in his patients led him to denounce the War on

Drugs as a failure in terms of policy and he argues for more compassion and creation of a safe, enriched environment.

Johann Hari interpreted the results of the Rat Park study in 2015 to assert that addiction is a likely consequence of failure of human connection. In his now popular TED Talk titled 'Everything you know about addiction is wrong', which has been watched close to 8 million times at the time of writing, he makes a passionate plea to view and change policy on addiction treatment.[20]

The reward pathway

You may be wondering how all this relates to opioids, pregabalin or gabapentin. It is time to view opioid addictions in a more compassionate light as well. I don't for a moment deny that opioids are addictive; they obviously act on the reward pathway. It is the same for gabapentin and pregabalin, which were reclassified as potentially addictive and therefore controlled drugs in 2019.

However, the lack of a stable environment that is less stressful and more supportive is often an equally important factor to address when deciding whether a drug could become more potent and a possible cause of addiction.

The reward system shown in the diagram on page 72 consists mainly of two brain structures called the ventral tegmental area (VTA) and the nucleus accumbens, and two chemicals called GABA and our internal opioids called the endorphins. As shown, many drugs, and in fact many other forms of 'addiction' (sugar/alcohol/nicotine and even porn and social media), all act on these structures in the brain. All of these reward the brain and make up for the lack of social connection and stress that is pervasive.

REWARD PATHWAY

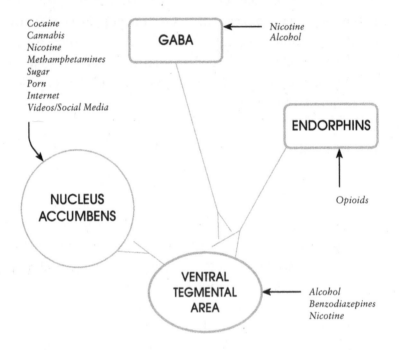

REWARD SYSTEM *Various drugs and substances act here*

So, the more important question to ask is not whether a particular pain-relief drug is more addictive or not, but whether you are at more risk of the drug acting more powerfully on your reward pathway than you think.

The opioid risk tool

In my clinical practice, I often use a scale called the 'opioid risk tool' before starting anyone on opioids.[21] This is a self-administered simple screening tool developed in 2005 by Dr Lynn Webster, and it takes less than a minute to do.

Mark each box that applies	Female	Male
Family history of substance abuse		
Alcohol	1	3
Illegal drugs	2	3
Prescription drugs	4	4
Personal history of substance abuse		
Alcohol	3	3
Illegal drugs	4	4
Prescription drugs	5	5
Age between 16 and 45 years old	1	1
History of preadolescent sexual abuse	3	0
Psychological disease		
Attention deficit disorder, bipolar, schizophrenia, obsessive compulsive disorder	2	2
Post-traumatic stress disorder, depression	1	1
Score Total		

A score of 3 or lower suggests a low risk for future opioid abuse. A score of 4 to 7 indicates moderate risk, and a score of 8 or greater indicates a high risk for abuse. If you score 4 or above, please discuss with your GP/specialist the risks and benefits of trialling any potentially dependence-inducing drug. If you are already on a strong opioid and scored more than 4 and you feel ready to reduce or taper the drug with support, then contact your GP/specialist to discuss your options.

Coming Off Your Medication

One of the biggest problems with any pain relief medication is the side effect risk, and many people want to reduce their drugs because of the perceived risk of becoming dependent on them. I think you should actively think about tapering or reducing your medications if:

- They are not clinically useful.
- The side effects are not tolerable or worse than the benefits.
- You are worried about dependence issues.
- The reason for taking it has gone away, either because the pain settled on its own or you had surgery or some other more targeted medication.

Betsan Corkhill, a well-being and lifestyle health coach, works with patients in a community setting. She highlights a few important points that patients often tell her they are worried about. See how much they apply to you:

- A conflict between wanting to come off and being afraid of not having any alternatives.
- Fears about side effects but afraid to voice these fears because 'the doctor might take me off my meds'.
- Confusions because of different opinions from different professionals.

- Worrying, one-sided reports in media about the drugs.
- Feeling alone, very scared, completely unsupported over the longer term.
- Not knowing the reasons for taking the medications so not adhering to the schedules.
- Lack of good, accessible, convenient, viable alternatives.
- Feelings of shame and failure because they are on so many medications.

Reducing or coming off your medication is a very difficult decision to make. Below are some broad suggestions to support you, but it's important to work with your GP/specialist to identify what is important to you so they can help you make the right decision regarding switching you to another better/ safer medication or reducing and stopping the drug.

T: Tenderness	Be kind and compassionate to yourself. Ensure that you have family/friends/loved ones to support you through the plan. All the worries mentioned above can happen and that's normal.
A: Addiction is not the same as dependence	Dependence and withdrawal are likely to happen, but are not to be feared and are not addiction. Discuss this with your specialist/GP if needed.
P: Pros and cons	Weigh up the pros and cons of the decision to taper. Think of what it will mean to you and your life and safety/functional improvement, and if it is worth it.
E: Embrace other strategies	Be ready to implement other mind–body strategies like mindfulness and exercise, as outlined in this book.

R: Rate of reduction	Start small and go slow. Aim to reduce by 10 per cent weekly if it is an opioid. Always discuss this with your pharmacist/GP/ specialist.

The Placebo Effect

Understanding the placebo effect and its evil twin, the nocebo response (see page 78), has been a great advance in managing pain and, if you know how to harness it effectively, can be of great help in reducing your pain. This is a powerful tool in your pain-free mindset toolbox.

A placebo is generally thought of as any drug or treatment that has no potential therapeutic value. Any scientific drug study is always done by comparing the drug to a placebo and, if we can show that it works better than the placebo, the drug is often approved. This is because we know that, although the placebo may have just been a sugar pill, it does have a noticeable effect in the brain – this is called the 'placebo effect'.

When I was in medical school, placebos always had a bit of a bad press and were considered unethical by some doctors. However, that has changed significantly in recent years due to our better understanding of the way the placebo effect occurs. We now know that the placebo effect is not just the sugar pill alone – it is all the various interactions that the patient receives from the professional/GP/specialist: the care, attention, the communication and the rapport. In fact, Harvard professor of medicine Ted Kaptchuk did a study on patients with IBS and showed that even when you tell patients that they are going to get a placebo (called an open-label), they still get a benefit.[22]

The most interesting public demonstration of the placebo effect for back pain was broadcast on BBC2 in 2018. This was led by Dr Michael Mosley, who conducted Britain's largest ever study called 'Opticare' into the placebo effect.[23] All 117 patients from Blackpool had long-term back problems and they were invited to be part of a trial for a new pain medication – a blue/white pill placed in a proper authentic bottle containing 120 tablets each having a strength of 400mg to be taken twice a day. They were told that some of them would get a placebo while others would get the new drug. One group had a standard GP consultation of less than 10 minutes while the other group had 30 minutes with an empathetic GP who listened to their pain problems before dispensing the new drug or placebo.

One of the patients they interviewed was 71-year-old Jim Pearce who at the beginning of the study was wheelchair bound, and on morphine and ketamine for his back pain. He had a desire to get back on his riverboat that he had to give up because of his pain.

Three weeks later when Dr Mosley and his team went back to see how they were doing, an astonishing thing had happened. More than half of the patients had a medically significant improvement in their pain. Jim had come off his entire morphine and was only on the 'powerful' new blue/white pills. He had also come out of the wheelchair and was able to get into the riverboat.

He, along with all the others, was given the results. They were informed that they had all been given a placebo. No one had received any new drug. Even after knowing this, most of them still preferred to be on the new drug despite knowing that it didn't have anything other than ground-rice within the capsule. Such is the power of the mind when needed.

What Mosley demonstrated here was the power of the placebo effect in reducing pain without the side effects and with all the benefits. What is becoming very clear is that a placebo can be as effective as a traditional treatment in many pain conditions. There is more chemical process going on than just positive thinking and there are now areas identified in the brain where this effect is processed.

It is now thought that the driving force behind the various experiments, including Mosley's Blackpool one, is the simple act and ritual of taking a pill and doing a certain action in a consistent fashion. That in itself becomes a positive healing practice. One way of giving yourself a placebo is the practice of various rituals and habits of healthy living: the right diet, a regular exercise pattern and therapies for the whole person (mind and body). These can all be part of the ingredients of the placebo effect and are all discussed in later chapters. At the level of the brain and spinal cord, placebos release the same chemicals that would be released when you take an actual drug. Good communication, trust and expectations of benefit will amplify the placebo response and increase the internal release of the body's own endorphins. They seem to work best on those who are open to the idea of new experiences and have a growth mindset – the willingness to learn a new thing. Would you consider taking a placebo knowing it might help?

The nocebo response

Let us start with the word itself. It means in Latin 'I shall harm' and refers to the negative expectations of any particular event, drug or treatment that then ends up making it more painful.

If I told you about a drug and its benefits and side effects and emphasised in great detail the possible bad side effects then there is a much higher chance that you might experience those side effects. That is the nocebo response.[24]

Likewise, we now understand that the language that we doctors and healthcare professionals use in describing some things about a drug or your condition can make you quite anxious and worried, and all of that will mean it can increase the side effects or even reduce the effects of any treatment.

At a clinical level, once you experience the side effects to a drug because of those negative expectations you will not want to take the drug. Physiologically, it causes your body to release chemicals and hormones like cortisol, which will amplify those initial feelings and strengthen them for future use. It can then impact how you react to other drugs from the same group as well.

ASSESS YOUR PAIN MEDICATION

Make a list of all your meds, those that you have tried and what side effects you have had, and those that you haven't tried at all.

- What are your present pain-relief medications?
- Name the non-steroids you have tried and those that you are on.
- Write down the names of any nerve tablets you are on.
- Write down the names of any strong opioids you are on.
- Write down the names of any other drugs you believe are for pain or muscle relaxation.
- What worrying beliefs do you have about those drugs that you are on?
- Are you worried about the drug's problems and side effects?

- Do you know someone who has had problems with these drugs and is that a reason for you not being keen to take them or start new drugs?

If you are having other side effects to pain medications or other drugs then you can go to rxisk.org, which aims to educate and inform about side effects to help your discussion with your specialist. Another useful resource is askapatient.com. If you want to look at other patient stories around medications then check out painkillers dontexist.com.

Take all this info to your doctor so that it becomes a proper discussion and you are as informed as you can be about what you can do/want to do regarding medications.

Summary

- There are a wide variety of pain medications that can help your pain. However, medications only work well when there is proven nociception.
- In the absence of nociception, medications don't work effectively.
- The NNT and NNH are useful ways to know if a drug is worth trying or not.
- Addiction is always a risk with the stronger medications because they act on the reward pathway in your brain.
- Whether you become addicted or not depends on your social support or connection and not on the drug itself.
- There are ways to manage the pain without drugs, which we'll cover in later chapters.

CHAPTER 4

Interventions

The most rewarding aspect of being a surgeon is watching patients go pain-free without surgery.

David Hanscom, spine surgeon

TINA HAS NOW suffered with low back pain for more than ten years. I got to know her through her work on social media and her blog where she writes extensively about her experiences of dealing with her pain. She also talks about the encounters she has had with various healthcare professionals and explores what patients would actually want from clinicians.

Her pain is very typical of how back pain starts in a large part of the population: 'My pain started quite suddenly. It was basically a manual handling injury. I had been cleaning out a Victorian house loft for a couple of weeks prior to it starting. The pain started on a Saturday morning. I had woken up with no pain or difficulties and my husband and I decided to go out for coffee at a local beauty spot. As I sat in the car, I could feel a little bit of a niggle, but by the time I came home at lunchtime, I just knew that there was something really wrong. By the end of the day, I couldn't walk. The next day, my husband called our GP and I was put on painkillers, but the pain continued. On the following day, I realised I hadn't passed urine for 24 hours and was unable to do so.'

Suspecting a pinching of the spinal cord (cauda equina), Tina was admitted to the local hospital for five days and a MRI scan found that there was a prolapsed disc 'compressing on the sciatic nerve root'. It took four to five weeks before she could start to walk and she said, 'Sitting down was impossible for weeks and weeks and, even now, to be honest, sitting down is quite painful for me. In the beginning, getting dressed was difficult. I couldn't make a meal and I had to have quite a lot of support to be able to function day to day. It's been a gradual improvement since that time.'

Over the next year Tina had high levels of pain medication, physiotherapy and guided injections – a nerve block and four caudal (tail bone) injections into the spine – and finally she underwent surgery 17 months after the initial episode of pain. Unfortunately, even that did not work and she was left with a diagnosis of failed back surgery. As she said, 'I was treated biomedically (with medications/injections/surgery) for the first three or four years following my injury.' She was never even referred to a pain clinic.

Surgery is often considered as the definitive fix for all pains, especially when it comes to many forms of pain within orthopaedics, but it is also extended to other specialities like urology, general surgery or gynaecology. By 'interventions', I am referring to steroid/cortisone injections like nerve blocks and epidurals that are done by pain physicians like myself and surgeries offered by various surgeons.

As someone who has been trained to offer injections, I have to declare my conflict of interest. Steroid injections do work and I use them often, but only if I think there is inflammation. Much like medication, injections work best when there is a focus of nociception and, in this case, they have an important place in acute pain management.

However, interventions are wholly driven by the Cartesian model, which means that our entire assumption is that pain always starts from a peripheral structure, so if you can block it, cut it, numb it or remove it, then there shouldn't be any pain. This is a very biomedical approach.

As we saw in Chapter 1, nociception is very different from pain (see page 20). If there is no nociception or little of it then the injection or surgery isn't going to be as effective as you or the clinician might hope. At least with injections of steroid, there is less risk of harm and less risk of permanent damage when compared to surgery. Nevertheless, they don't have any long-term benefits and often have to be repeated, which is now coming under a lot of scrutiny from insurers/NHS commissioners.

Every week, I have at least 10 patients amongst the 25 to 30 who I see who are convinced that surgery will take away their pain and they can't see the point of seeing me, trying medications or injections and wasting their time, my time and even the time of the NHS. We have been almost conditioned to believe in the complete effectiveness of surgery of every kind. We think any new way of doing surgery must be better than an old way and that the longer the duration or complexity, the more important it must be and that 'the doctor would not recommend an operation unless it was effective and in the best interests of the patient'.

That is unfortunately not true at all. As Ian Harris, professor of orthopaedic surgery at the University of New South Wales, Australia, boldly proclaimed: 'the placebo effect is one of the factors contributing to the overestimation of the true effectiveness of surgery'.[1]

One of the problems is that many physicians have not fully understood the person in pain before subjecting them to major surgery. For example, most patients going for joint replacement surgery have varying degrees of preoperative pain. We now have evidence that central sensitisation (see page 53) can occur with osteoarthritis.[2] This means that there does not need to be nociception at the affected joint (no active chemicals being released) but there will still be a perceived pain due to central sensitisation in the spinal cord and brain. It stands to reason, therefore, that injections of steroid and even surgery are not likely to be fully successful in these patients.

Very few hospitals in the UK, either on the NHS or privately, actively try to address and improve on these preoperative factors before recommending surgery. Increasingly, I see patients whose pain hasn't changed due to surgery or has got worse. There are often multiple reasons and, in almost all these cases, there is very little nociception and increasing pain experience and central sensitisation. I have also become more careful with who I give injections to these days.

Ben's story

Ben was referred to me in 2010. In his twenties he worked as a DJ for a local radio station. He created chilled-out jazz and lounge music and that style of music-making was also reflected in his genial personality.

His pain started after a bad viral infection when he was interning in his teens. He was left with chronic pain and fatigue. Once the fatigue had started to settle down, he noticed an intense burning pain that went down both his legs. He described it as 'a constant feeling of scalding burning water poured down my legs'.

He was seeing one of my colleagues and spent about six to eight years trying a variety of nerve blocks and epidurals for his pain with no obvious long-term relief. To me it looked like a case of complex regional pain syndrome (CRPS). This can be a very tricky problem to solve for many patients and NICE recommends consideration of spinal cord stimulation (SCS) for conditions like Ben's.

SCS is a more high-tech form of transcutaneous electrical nerve stimulation (TENS) machines where a fine wire is placed through an epidural needle on top of the spinal cord. The needle is then removed and the wire is connected to a pacemaker-like box that can deliver electrical impulses that generate a more acceptable throbbing or pulsing that gets preferentially sent to the brain. The brain then decides that it likes the throbbing sensation rather than the nociception from the surgical area and that accounts for reduced pain perception. It isn't a fix, but it's an excellent distraction technique that blocks and modifies the signals that may be coming from a peripheral source. In Ben's case, we still did not have a clear idea of where the pain was being generated, though I suspected it could have been the spinal cord. Ben had the SCS and it changed his life and improved his pain considerably.

There are several success stories of people like Ben where procedures like this and other major surgeries make a great difference. However, unfortunately the story doesn't end there. Poor Ben ended up getting an infection and that meant that the implant (pacemaker box) had to come out.

There we were, once again, on a cool December morning in my clinic: 'Is this how it's going to be, Doc? I want to be pain-free, but I just don't see more surgery as a good option going forward. Getting injections every three months? It just hasn't been kind to me. The SCS itself has been brilliant, but the infection hasn't.'

The Problem with Interventions

Seeing what happened to Ben and Tina – and many of the other patients I have looked after and learnt from – really opened my eyes to the efficacy of injections and surgery and led me to ask more fundamental questions of what we think interventions really achieve and what is possible for patients when the intervention hasn't worked.

At the end of the day it is important to ask: Where do interventions and surgery play a part in pain management and what do patients and surgeons/clinicians want? All patients in pain want to be free from pain and they assume erroneously that since the problem comes from a structure, removing that structure should take away that problem. That seems straightforward enough, but with the complexity of pain and the number of structures likely to be playing a part, it is a wrong starting place for many patients.

Surgeons want to do a good job and avoid infection or complications. What I think is missing is the assessment of the person in pain at the time of going for surgery because everyone feels that the problem is purely structural.

Often when it comes to conditions like arthritis of the knee or hip, the core belief of both patients and doctors/ surgeons is that surgery is inevitable. While I can understand that some emergency situations – like the removal of an appendix or an acute disc prolapse causing weakness of legs and/or incontinence – need surgery, most of the other patients are often operated on because of this belief.

Sometimes surgeons are dismissive of more conservative approaches, while at other times they might feel that the patient would not adhere to exercise and conservative models of pain management, but these are all personal biases as a result of not keeping up to date with changing evidence or a refusal to accept it as it conflicts with the way they think about the problem.

While a lot of the data below may be related to orthopaedic surgery, as often these patients are the largest number of people referred to pain clinics, in my experience this principle applies to all surgeons in all specialities. Professor Ian Harris identifies a few broad themes:[3]

The post hoc fallacy

The post hoc fallacy is a false belief that most of us, including doctors and surgeons, subscribe to. Essentially, it is the assumption that if a particular event X happened after an event Y then we automatically assume that X was caused by Y. For example, if we were to think that every time the rooster crows the sun comes up, that would be an example of a post hoc fallacy.[4]

With pain, this is very common. If we get an episode of neck or lower back pain, we then get a scan done and it might show signs of disc bulging or disc dehydration. While these are perfectly normal events that happen (just like grey hair as we get older), because the scan was done after an episode of pain, the disc bulge is then said to be responsible for that pain. This then drives further treatment and investigations.

Now it may be true that scans would pick up a tumour or growth on some occasions, which could very well explain the reason for pain, but in most of orthopaedics, the chances are much higher that the changes were already there before the pain or the scan happened.

NORMAL FINDINGS ON SCAN

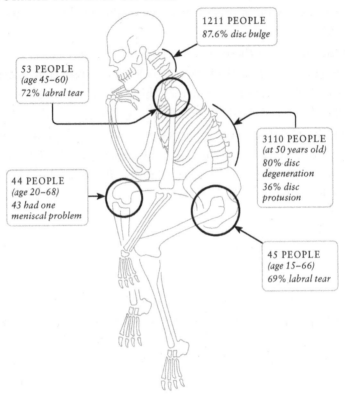

1211 PEOPLE
87.6% disc bulge

53 PEOPLE
(age 45–60)
72% labral tear

3110 PEOPLE
(at 50 years old)
80% disc
degeneration
36% disc
protusion

44 PEOPLE
(age 20–68)
43 had one
meniscal problem

45 PEOPLE
(age 15–66)
69% labral tear

The diagram above shows the studies that have been done on different joints of the body. What is remarkable is these changes in structure occur in these parts of the body, for example in the hip, knee, shoulder or back, and are often there for many years before any pain actually occurs. Sometimes there is never any pain and these are discovered quite by chance.

The astonishing thing is that these studies have all been done in patients who have essentially got no symptoms but their X-rays or MRIs all show changes of age-related degeneration. We can see from this that surgery can often be unnecessary.

In my opinion, the post hoc fallacy has been the main reason for continued over-medicalisation and overzealous interventions and surgeries. When I referred Ben for the surgery or the SCS, I believed that it might actually solve the problem. I think a lot of surgeons recommend the operations thinking they are also doing the right thing. However, after five years of reading through the scientific literature, I have seen that sometimes the evidence for surgery is just not there; much of the time the strength of evidence supporting the surgery is weak or it has been proven not to be good or the harms are much worse. Things are improving now and professor of orthopaedic surgery Ian Harris makes a claim for doing more research to critically ask which of our existing surgeries work and are good value for the patient and society at large.

The flawed belief in society

The post hoc fallacy combines with a related but different belief that injections and more invasive options like surgery are always successful. Though these may be extreme options, they are always perceived as a fix so are then considered to be the final option that will always be paid for and supported and understood by everyone in society.

As I have said before, surgery certainly may be the right thing if you need to have your appendix removed, a baby delivered or a tumour/cyst/growth taken out, but it does not mean that the pain is only from that area. Even with cysts and some tumours, the same principle applies that sometimes these are discovered when you are being investigated for something else and therefore have nothing to do with your pain. There is no correlation between the intensity of pain and the size of the tumour or cyst.

Lack of knowledge dissemination

As a member of the public, you assume to a great extent that a doctor or surgeon knows what they're doing. However, pain is incredibly complex and understanding the distinction between nociception and pain is not something your surgeon/specialist would necessarily be aware of. Most UK specialists in their forties might have received an average of 12 hours of pain education in five to seven years of medical school.[5] What we would have been taught is the Cartesian biomedical approach where often removal of a part is expected to result in relief of pain as the solution.

Lack of good regulation

There is another problem with surgical implants and studies related to them. Usually drugs are very rigorously tested on animals and then humans before being made available for the general public. However, there is no such requirement for a surgical technique or implant to be subjected to the same kind of discipline before it is marketed to the surgeons and public. This is starting to change, but a lot of the problems that have been reported with breast implants, metal hip replacements and vaginal meshes were because of a lack of regulation and proper research into long-term safety.

No incentive to change

Since it works some of the time there is often no incentive to change practice. If there is good relief for a short term (a few months), then it still validates the technique so there is no reason to change what we do. That is often at odds with what you as the patient want.

When surgeries are introduced, it is often on the 'wobbly tripod of evidence' as Harris calls it:[6]

1. There is a biological explanation that sounds logical and plausible ('There is a disc that looks like it is touching the nerve on the scan, so if I can take it out, the patient's pain will go away').
2. 'I have seen or read about it working in the lab or in a few animals therefore it should work in this human.'
3. 'I have done it before or have seen my mentor do it before and it worked so it should work.'

All of these are flaws in critical thinking. Surgery and interventions of any kind, whether they are for spinal, orthopaedic, pelvic, urology or gynaecological surgery, all suffer from the same biases and outcomes. The painful truth is that surgery has never been trialled or compared to a sham surgical approach (placebo) to see if it truly makes a difference. However, in the last 10 to 20 years this has changed.

A number of surgeries have now been tested against a sham surgery. For example, a group of Dutch researchers took 180 people above the age of 50 with vertebral (back bone) fractures.[7] They all had significant pain and loss of function. Ninety-one of these patients received vertebroplasty (a surgery that involved injecting cement into the bones of the spine for osteoporosis-related fracture). Eighty-nine patients went off to sleep, but they did not get the actual injection of cement, just the tiny cuts on the outside and some local anaesthetic near the bone as a pretend anaesthesia (a sham surgery).

PLACEBO SURGERIES BY AREA

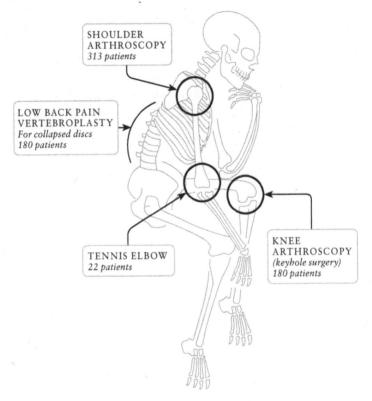

SHOULDER
ARTHROSCOPY
313 patients

LOW BACK PAIN
VERTEBROPLASTY
For collapsed discs
180 patients

TENNIS ELBOW
22 patients

KNEE
ARTHROSCOPY
(keyhole surgery)
180 patients

The patients were followed at 1 month and then at 12 months after the procedure. Both groups had more than a 50 per cent improvement in pain by 1 month and it was maintained at 12 months, and there was no difference between the groups. Now you might say that the whole ritual of coming to a hospital and going off to sleep all made a difference and you could be right. But in the sham group, we could get the same benefit without any of the side effects of the dangerous cement injection.

Dr Adriaan Louw, an expert pain science educator and author of the book *Pain Neuroscience Education*, reviewed all the areas of the body where surgery was done in comparison to sham procedures (placebo) in 2017. Sham surgery trials had been done for low back pain, knee pain, shoulder pain, osteoporosis-related spine pain and tennis elbow. His team found that in every one of them there was no difference between the placebo and the actual surgery![8]

All surgeries have risks of infection and of causing some nerve damage or worsening the pain. When they don't work, it causes more distress to the patient. The surgeon might then feel compelled on some occasions to offer a repeat or addition.

Post-Surgical Pain

In the table below you will see that most surgeries have a high risk of leaving you with chronic pain afterwards.[9] For example, up to 20 per cent of patients undergoing knee replacements are going to have a different kind of pain that will still leave them with poor quality of life and possibly on medication.[10] Often these are the very reasons for people with osteoarthritis going for surgery.

Kind of surgery	Percentage risk of post-surgical pain
Knee replacement	13–44%
Hip replacement	27%
Breast surgery (mastectomy)	11–57%
Caesarean section	6–55%

Amputation	30–85%
Gall bladder removal	3–50%
Abdominal surgery	17–21%
Inguinal hernia repair	5–63%
Hysterectomy	32%
Spine surgery	20%

At the outset, let us define two types of surgery-related pain:

The first is where you might have a certain pain for which you think that surgery is the next or only or final option. This might be for conditions like osteoarthritis, an appendix, bladder- or bowel-related surgery, back pain or neck pain. As a pain physician I often see many patients whose chronic pain persists despite technically adequate surgery.

The second is the group of patients where I think nerve damage has happened during surgery and we call that 'post-surgical neuropathic pain'.

Could you have post-surgical neuropathic pain?[11]

- Is your pain still present and has it been more than three months after surgery?
- Was there any pain similar to this before surgery?
- Does this pain feel different to the pain you had before surgery?
- Is it localised to the area of surgery?

If you have answered 'Yes' to all of the above then it is likely that you have post-surgical neuropathic pain.

It is now thought that the pain in these situations is more complex and will be a combination of some nociception from the site of surgery (scars, etc.) but also hypersensitivity in the spinal cord or brain pathways (a kind of inflammation in the immune cells throughout the nervous system that is different to our usual understanding and treatment for inflammation).

It is well known that the following can all increase the risk of having an unsuccessful outcome after any surgery:[12]

- If you have chronic pain in the same area.
- If you have multiple medical problems.
- If you have ongoing mental health issues like anxiety and depression.

When surgery goes wrong

There are several problems that can arise when surgery goes wrong:

- Psychological: Failed surgery can cause psychological issues, leaving the patient recovering from the first failed surgery and the rehabilitation time. Facing the uncertainty of going through it all again can lead to anxiety and worry.
- Financial: Financially, someone (the patient, insurer or the NHS) will now have to pay for a second surgery. In addition, the extra time off could have an effect on the patient's return to work or productivity for a family.
- Harm: A failed surgery, or one with complications, can cause significant harm and excessive mortality and morbidity, and if surgery was unnecessary to start with then it needs to be investigated and reviewed.

To me, the harm failed surgery causes is the worst problem. Often this is a concern that is not on either the surgeon's or the patient's mind, but we've all seen the headlines in recent years around the problems of metal hip replacements and, more recently, the vaginal mesh repair issues.

What if the surgery may have never been needed in the first instance? Could we be barking up the wrong tree?

Why Do People Still Want Surgery?

There are multiple reasons why people still want to go ahead with surgery.

Desire to do something

Often it becomes a collective group hug where both the patient and doctors feel that surgery is a typical way to solve the problem. A patient may not feel comfortable with the idea of 'Is this my life now?' I have had some younger patients tell me with some frustration, 'I am only 26. I won't let this beat me. I am going to do what it takes to be pain-free, even if that means multiple surgeries!'

Nocebo language

The second issue is, once a structural change has been picked up on the scan or X-ray, surgeons often then end up giving their personal opinions on this. At this point, they might introduce nocebos, which can often worry patients considerably (see page 78).

In my own practice, I have had a 65-year-old lady once tell me that she wouldn't do any exercise because her surgeon had told her about her right knee being 'bone on bone' on the scan, and that she needed the surgery as soon as possible otherwise it could affect the hip and back. He had cautioned her against doing any activity as it could make it worse.

Another was a gentleman in his sixties who was flippantly warned by his surgeon that had he delayed his arrival any longer, he would have ended up in a wheelchair in a couple of months as his spine was 'crumbling'. His comments on the man's X-ray being the worst the surgeon had seen in his practice also compounded the patient's worry and depression.

Most human beings are visual learners. Statements like the above are often interpreted by the patient's brain with very disturbing but powerful visual images. Those images then stick and it can often be very hard to undo such a belief and surgery is perceived as the only course of action. What healthcare professionals say has an enduring influence on patients' beliefs – when researchers asked 130 people about their chronic low back pain and where their wrong beliefs came from, 89 per cent said that they had got them from a healthcare professional.[13]

Approved by insurers or the NHS

What is not often articulated in the NHS for fear of being seen as rationing care is the cost of these surgeries. Drs Vinay Prasad and Adam Cifu, American medical doctors and world-class researchers, in their book *Ending Medical Reversal*, and Professor Ian Harris, Australian orthopaedic surgeon, in *Surgery, the Ultimate Placebo*, cite a variety of doctor- or surgeon-related factors for continuing to keep operating or investigating despite the mounting evidence against common surgeries.[14]

They suggest that the way many healthcare systems are built and paid for is by the number of surgeries that are done. This payment by numbers was actually the way the NHS also set up contracts until 2017–18 and it has only changed since early 2019. Now the evidence is being reviewed more critically and a lot of injections and surgeries that were being offered routinely on the NHS are being decommissioned or not being paid for anymore.

I think with the right kind of rehabilitation support there is still a role for interventions in carefully chosen patients who are optimised. However, the evidence is still not adequate to convince the insurers and NHS.

Is An Intervention Right For You?

Choosing Wisely is an international group supported by multiple governments to enable patients to think about their treatment options more carefully.[15] They recommend that all patients ask the following four questions – forming the acronym BRAN – when discussing future surgeries with their specialists:

What are the **B**enefits?

- What do you understand about the benefits of the proposed surgery?
- Has it been explained to you?
- What benefits should you get and how long will it take?
- Do these benefits match what outcomes you want?

Often there is a subtle but very important distinction between what the surgeon thinks is an ideal outcome and what you would like. Make sure that you are both on the same page. If you and the surgeon jointly think that the surgery is going to achieve your desired outcome, then go ahead. Otherwise, be fully prepared to have a longer discussion with them to know the exact risks and outcomes.

What are the Risks?

- Have the risks been explained to you?
- Do you understand what the risks mean in simple terms?

There can often be a communication gap between what doctors say and what patients hear. This difference can be best appreciated when doctors explain risk. Sometimes it is so vague that patients cannot understand. This concept of informed consent has become very important and, after a major court victory in 2015, it became clear that what is important for the patient as a rational person is that they should be told of all risks and benefits so that they can make the appropriate decision.

You may debate whether a patient can deem to know everything and be in a position to challenge a healthcare professional, but my view is that with chronic-pain-related surgical plans, the advances in pain have been so significant that it is more likely that you would know your pain and understand it much better than most healthcare professionals. Therefore it is up to you to take that active interest to make sure that the risks are worth the benefits, because no surgery or any injections, even the ones that I do and that a lot of my colleagues will be doing, are ever free from risk or are proven to be a guaranteed success in all patients.

What are the **A**lternatives?

- Have suitable alternatives been explained to you?
- Were you given information about the various alternatives to surgery?
- Was there any suggestion of various resources and signposting to other options that could be looked at if surgery wasn't going to be an option or wasn't a safe enough option?

Since the guarantee for surgery is virtually non-existent, you should be informed of the alternatives to any interventional procedure that can cause harm and these should be explored with you.

If your surgeon is not aware of the details of any alternative treatments to give an unbiased impartial understanding, you may have to seek the support of your GP or pain specialist to explore the alternatives to surgery. If you still feel that surgery represents a huge opportunity, then go ahead.

It is important to optimise your general health before you go for surgery. Ensure that you get a significant period of prehabilitation (to get ready for surgery in terms of the mind and body) and find other ways of learning to do things and look after yourself as you recover, which could mean learning some of the skills of self-care. It is better that you practise this before surgery so that it becomes easier to do after surgery, than to start something new afterwards.

What if I do **N**othing?

This is often a very important but underappreciated question and it is about having an open mind. My colleague once told me about a 75-year-old elderly pensioner, Mr Smith, who had started to experience some 'niggles' and pains in his left hip for a few weeks. Fast-forward to some imaging that showed suggestions of hip osteoarthritis and a chat with his GP. After one physio visit led to another, he found himself in front of a surgeon who said that they could offer to resurface the hip to 'sort' the problem. This was the procedure Andy Murray underwent so that he could return to playing tennis.

The patient had a mild neurological condition and his neurologist had warned him that any surgery could risk his neurological condition becoming worse. My anaesthetic colleague saw this person in a preoperative assessment prior to his surgery a week later.

Mr Smith was in a state of confusion because of this conflicting advice from the surgeon to get the surgery done and from the neurologist who warned differently. My colleague expertly, patiently and, more importantly, compassionately explored this in some detail. She informed him about the time taken for recovery and rehabilitation usually required after a hip replacement in terms of physio and exercises. At that time, Mr Smith remarked that he was able to spend two hours in the garden most days and that he still had a decent night's sleep if he took some paracetamol. He was still independent and able to drive to the high street to do the shopping.

He asked my colleague what if he just did nothing and carried on. My colleague helped him make this decision and ran through what that would look like and what he might have to do to keep active. He did exactly that and thanked my colleague for helping him arrive at that plan.

Mr Smith didn't need the surgery, but what hadn't been explored with him was the fact that one *can* choose to do nothing. Our desire to be perceived as *doing* is a very human tendency, and doctors and surgeons are no different from any other member of the public.

The Holistic View

We've now seen the major issues with interventions and medications in pain management. Once you understand the limitations and usefulness of these two important but often overused techniques, you can start to appreciate why it is important to be aware of newer and safer long-term strategies to overcome your pain. This is where the pain-free mindset comes in.

Tina, who we met at the start of the chapter, finally met a physiotherapist four years into her journey who established a connection with her that allowed her to understand the complexity of her pain experience.

As she recalled, 'I assumed that my pain was from an injured part of my body and that, if a clinician fixed that injured part, I'd be fine. He took a much more functional approach with me. If I'd had a stroke, I'd have somebody to rehabilitate me straight away, but I had to wait four years before my rehabilitation started. My previous physiotherapists had done the normal sort of core exercises and manual therapy. They had held up a model of the spine and told me about discs prolapsing but, actually, that doesn't really tell you very much does it? They probably thought that they were educating me. It wasn't what I really needed. I needed a more personalised approach. It sounds absolutely daft, but I needed somebody to point out to me that stress makes my pain worse and that working too hard makes my pain worse. I needed professional support to be able to understand what was going on with my body and what was increasing and decreasing my pain.'

Tina's pain had persisted despite interventions and surgery. The reasons could have been possible nerve damage following the discectomy but, as she notes, stress and anxiety made it worse, as did the fear of being on stronger medications for life.

The therapeutic alliance that she developed with her physiotherapist, together with the support from family and her new identity as patient expert, also helped significantly. She lost her teaching career but made significant changes to her life and now lives a life that is calmer, more stress-free and she 'values things in a different way'. Her blog and her work supporting other clinicians and patients have enabled her to take on a new identity of an expert patient advocate who can guide both the public and the professional.

In Ben's case, it was important for him to also address the other mind–body issues and he started to do more exercise and self-management with yoga and dog walks. His wife, a Pilates teacher and physiotherapist, helped and he practised meditation/mindfulness with his own brand of music. He was then able to completely stop his dependence on strong opiates. All of this allowed him to have a much more productive life. It is now possible for Ben to balance and manage his pain and therefore control and achieve all that he is doing as a DJ, a father, a good husband, and to be productive.

Pain still troubles him and I still see him once every four to six months, but this is not the same Ben that I first met in 2010. This is someone much happier, at peace, with a pain-free mindset and a plan to look after himself and live a full life.

If you are now rethinking the very idea of surgery or you feel that surgery was never on the table as an option for you then do not worry. You are now ready to move on to understanding the role and importance of other aspects of the pain-free mindset that you can implement in your life to overcome your pain. *The Pain-Free Mindset* empowers you to really understand the various ways that pain can be reduced and overcome rather than just hoping for a surgical fix or medical miracle. Patients just like you are now leading more fulfilling lives with better quality and are on fewer drugs with no surgery. It is possible, and it all starts with understanding the nervous system and the protective role of pain through evolution.

Summary

- Interventions can be either injections of steroids or major surgeries.
- Unlike drugs, most surgeries have never been tested against a control or placebo. When such studies have been done, there appears to be no benefit.
- Most surgeries have an element of risk of post-surgical chronic pain with no success.
- Interventions are most useful when combined with a good prehabilitation or post-surgical rehabilitation plan.
- Always conduct the BRAN test for any surgery or injection that you are going to have.

CHAPTER 5

Neuroscience and Stress Management

The biology of pain is never really straightforward, even when it appears to be.

Professor Lorimer Moseley, clinical scientist
and pain researcher

THIS BY FAR is the most important chapter for me and I hope it will be for you as well. The advances that have happened in our understanding of chronic pain have been made possible with fancy ways of seeing the functioning brain under a scan. Practising in the clinic seeing up to 50 patients a week in the hospital and community, these discoveries helped me to better understand patients like Debbie far better than I could have hoped.

Debbie's story

Debbie's pain problems started with a relatively innocent episode of acute low back pain at work about eight years ago. A scan at that time revealed a disc bulge. After being told that this was the reason for her pain, she underwent four sessions of NHS physiotherapy, which did not help her. After not getting much relief from an injection, she ended up with a discectomy in 2012. This unfortunately did not work completely so it left her with more persistent and intense low back pain with left-sided sciatica-like pain down her left leg.

She then complained of left knee pain, so after physiotherapy, was referred to the knee surgeon. She was recommended a keyhole (arthroscopy) surgery so that they could wash out her arthritic changes. That did not work so she was recommended a mini knee replacement in 2013. However, pain continued unabated.

Then she started to get shoulder pain. Guess what happened?

After not getting any benefit from physiotherapy and medications, she was referred to a shoulder surgeon and was diagnosed to have impingement, for which she had a keyhole washout of her shoulder (remember what I said about these surgeries in the last chapter?). It seemed to work for about three months and then the pain returned, not just in the operated shoulder but also in the other shoulder.

All this time, she was also seeing me in the pain clinic for her back pain. I initially did some joint injections followed by an epidural, neither of which helped for more than a few months. In the interim, she developed frequent headaches and was diagnosed as having migraine. The migraine drugs weren't particularly helpful. By this time, over a period of five years, her pains had become widespread so she saw a rheumatologist who diagnosed her with fibromyalgia. She was also diagnosed with IBS and an 'irritable bladder'.

Debbie was on codeine, co-codamol, naproxen, tramadol, strong opiates and nerve tablets, and all her symptoms and complaints stayed the same. Her notes ran to three volumes.

Does this strike a note with some of you? Have you had these multiple issues which seem to be present in many parts of the body? It began to dawn on me that I was seeing far too many patients like Debbie before surgery; some of them for day case procedures, some on inpatient ward rounds, others in outpatient clinics and community services, all with multiple, complex issues.

I wondered what we as healthcare professionals were doing wrong. What was the real problem? How can pain become so complex? Can someone have so many separate issues or could there be a common root cause?

This is something that has focused my attention for the last five years, trying to understand how to help such complex situations. First, I had to understand what was going on before I could figure out how I could help. This research led me to one tissue weighing three pounds. Actually, to be precise, two tissues/organs weighing about six pounds in total: the brain and then the second brain, the gut.

Some of the biggest advances in pain management that have occurred in the last 20 years have been in understanding more about the nervous system and its links with the immune system and the controller, the brain and the second brain (gut). This has not only revolutionised the field of pain management but also so many others within medicine.

With regards to pain management, our better understanding of the two brains and the way they can be changed with exposure to repeated painful signals is very useful. It is tremendously exciting to realise that we can influence them together or separately and overcome pain. At the same time, they both can cause unusual symptoms in many patients and this can be a clinical challenge.

Pain is fundamentally a biopsychosocial phenomenon, meaning that for every pain there is a biological element to it; it has an effect on our psychology and how we feel; and, finally, it influences how our social relationships affect us

THE BIOPSYCHOSOCIAL MODEL

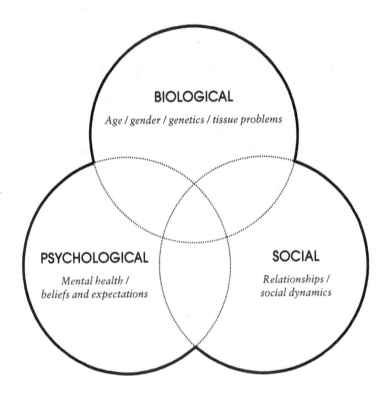

and our outlook towards the rest of society.[1] None of these can be separated from each other, but as you might have experienced in our healthcare system, most clinicians pay attention to the biology bit, but there is never much attention to the other two aspects.

With so much complexity and dependence on other factors, I would like to show you that:

- The brain tries to have a pre-prepared framework ready to predict danger.

- Because of this habit of prediction, nociception and pain often become very different.
- All the processes in the brain are geared to detect danger like an alarm system.
- It keeps learning by adapting and firing and wiring new circuits together.
- All parts of the brain are active in learning about danger and protecting so that it can predict better the next time.
- This is a whole-person (mind and body) effort to get it right, and the brain uses the vagus nerve and other stress mechanisms to try to keep you safe, sometimes at its own cost.

The Prediction Machine

The brain acts like a prediction machine – it has already created some predictions, based on previous experiences, on what would be a safe and quick way to respond to various situations we face in life. In the past, when our forefathers were hunter-gatherers and we were not sure where the sabre-toothed tiger was hiding, most quick reactions were more or less right in terms of safety.

However, in the modern world, though we don't have tigers, the system still thinks really fast as if it needs to protect you. If it gets the decision wrong and overprotects by amplifying the pain, then it stops being useful.

This prediction power of the brain can be best illustrated by two classic stories that were published in scientific journals. Both show opposite ends of the 'pain' spectrum.

A painful toenail

A 29-year-old construction worker was on a building site finishing his day's job when he suffered a freak accident. He jumped from a height on to a wooden plank and a seven-inch nail pierced his boot from the bottom and poked through the top.

Upon this happening, he was in such agony and was so upset that nothing could be done for him on site and he could not be consoled. With his pain worsening, an ambulance was called and he was taken to the nearest A&E. Once there, the doctors struggled to do anything to calm him down, despite the muscle relaxants and pain medications given both orally and intravenously.

Finally, the medical team gave him intravenous midazolam to sedate him and then pulled the nail out and took his boot off to examine and clean up the wound. To the utter surprise of the surgeons, they discovered that the nail had passed between the toes without even penetrating his skin. There was absolutely no damage to his skin or his toes and there was no blood or puncture wound.

Could you ever deny that the man was in pain? We couldn't say that he made it all up. If the worker saw this nail protruding from below and he had felt the nail piercing the boot then it was enough for his brain to activate safety mechanisms that would involve calling attention (crying and shouting in pain) and moving the foot very little (to decrease and quieten the pain).

This case report was published in 1995 and it demonstrates that the brain can perceive pain even when there is no injury.[2] In this example, there was no nociception but there was the pain experience.

Hitting the nail on the head

Construction workers have done their bit to improve our knowledge around pain management. Another construction worker was using a nail gun as part of his duties, when it accidentally and unexpectedly discharged, hitting him in the face.[3]

He had a mild toothache and developed a bruise under his jaw but didn't notice anything else. He must have counted his lucky stars and felt that he had had a narrow escape. He went about his daily work, continued to be fine and had no symptoms after that accident.

About a week later, he went to the dentist for a regular check-up. When an X-ray was done of his tooth, the radiographer and dentist were shocked that a four-inch nail was found embedded in his head. His dentist cross-questioned him regarding symptoms, but he was pain-free.

Something like that ought to have been painful and you might wonder if the worker was an outlier; maybe he had genes that caused him not to feel pain? But the reason is more exciting and hopeful.

Given the right environment, the brain can always be developed and changed to suit our needs. If we look at the predictive model of pain, we can see that there was nothing visual to guide the patient towards any seriousness until the X-ray was done.

Since the discharge of the nail gun was by nature a rare event, his brain did not have any predictions on what to look out for in terms of danger, so there was no danger signal or plan to amplify any pain. In this example, the worker had all the reasons for nociception but he had no pain.

There are many such stories that are often recounted online. The understanding that we have of our nervous system and the conclusions we then draw will sound very counter-intuitive to present teaching and thought. However, we are able to explain this a lot better using our understanding of the brain and how the nerve and immune pathways work and what they are designed for. Irrespective of the medical speciality, the most important aspect again bears repeating: *pain is never an accurate indicator of the degree of damage to your tissues or bones in the body.*

The stories above indicate that you can experience severe pain when there's no injury and no pain when there should really have been a significant amount of pain because the prediction maps are not the same.

The Protection Machine

The writer Paul Ingraham has identified up to 34 separate causes of pain and has looked at certain basic mechanisms or processes that can affect the nervous system.[4] While it shows that the system is complex, there are some common characteristics of most persistent pain, and understanding this is important because it reveals that this perception of pain is driven by a purpose to protect.

Nociception and pain are not the same

I know I have said it before, but nociception is the biological sensation of chemicals released when the nerves get a noxious (unpleasant) sensation. These chemicals then travel within the nerves and this is called nociception, which travels to the brain.

Pain, on the other hand, is what you *feel*. We often think that the severity of that pain is because of more damage or more inflammation, but this isn't the case. What you feel and how severe it feels is often entirely based on what your brain decides it should be based on and how much protection it needs to create – and this includes many other factors, such as context, prior experience and prediction.

That is a very important difference to understand. Many specialists do scans or tests and tell patients that their knee or back or neck are fine, but patients do not understand why their pain feels so severe (remember Elizabeth from Chapter 1).

I have at least one or two patients every week who say, 'I've been to more than three rheumatologists and two spinal surgeons and a pain consultant and so many physio sessions. I still can't understand why they didn't find anything wrong with me. Something has to be causing my pain and I need you to get to the bottom of it. Can I have another scan?'

Nociception always occurs. For every such experience, chemicals are released and signals are sent to the brain for interpretation. But for pain to be felt, the brain needs to be conscious and involved to decide on the intensity and severity.

For example, when you are under a general anaesthetic for surgery, the cut of the knife can cause your heart rate or blood pressure to go up, which is due to the nociceptive signal, but you don't feel any pain (and if you do then your anaesthetist isn't doing their job!).

Pain is the ultimate alarm system

Pain is a fundamental alarm system. That is what evolution designed it for – a warning or danger signal that there might be potential threat to life. It is excellent most of the time, but it can be overprotective and become maladaptive.

Dr Henry Beecher, a famous American anaesthetist during the Second World War, was one of the first to note that there was no correlation between the wound and the pain experienced: 'The intensity of suffering is largely determined by what the pain means to the patient.' In his study from 1956 comparing 150 soldiers to civilian patients, only 32 per cent of soldiers who had extensive wounds asked for opioids, while 83 per cent of the civilians requested them.[5]

We have gone through more than 50 years still looking for a biological and structural cause without paying attention to the importance of what pain means to the patient. In Beecher's study, it is likely that the soldiers would have considered the frontline of war to be a constant real danger. However, once they got injured and were admitted to hospital, that would be considered safety so there would be no need for the danger system to be that active. Interestingly, the same soldiers would considerably wince and express their disappointment in sometimes colourful language when given their injections by the nurses.

Our brain will create the experience of pain when it perceives a threat, regardless of whether tissue damage occurs or not.

The pain system is like the stress system. Ideally, the fight or flight response in stress should come on when there is danger to life, but we know that modern day-to-day issues and other non-life-threatening events, like a bad boss or a difficult child, can still be big stressors and activate the fight or flight response and, more importantly, activate and sensitise the immune system in our brain.

Similarly, the nociceptive system can become triggered even when there is no obvious reason to be, and certainly the brain can then amplify the entire experience – sometimes based on perception and sometimes on very few actual signals – indicating that it has become oversensitive. But that doesn't mean that you need to be given a strong opioid, an injection or surgery every time.

Neural Networks

When a nociceptive signal arrives at various parts of the brain, it activates the nerves in that area and then the brain learns from that experience and forms a network of nerves that helps it remember what to do the next time.

NEURAL NETWORK / NEUROTAGS

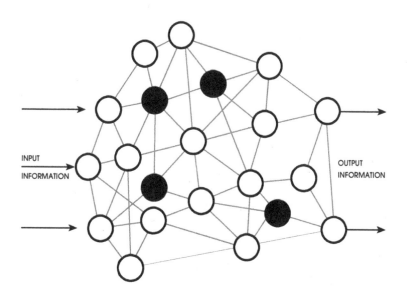

Lorimer Moseley and David Butler are world-famous pain researchers who have made it their lives' work to research this and teach other healthcare professionals. They put forward the theory of the 'neurotag' – a group of nerve cells that are linked with each other to form a group/network.[6] There are many such groups in the brain and often nerve cells from one network will also belong to another. They may either be helping with an action (action neurotags) or modifying another function (modulating neurotags).

Imagine if you are a working mum with two kids. You would have a social circle where you are part of different WhatsApp/Facebook groups – one group of your friends, another from your workplace and also, as is common these days, the parents from your kids' schools and their friends. Similarly, in the brain, neurons, like you, would be part of multiple networks.

If you are affected in some way and need help, that would have an impact on all the groups you are part of. Most (you hope) would change to support you; others, like your close friends or family members, may also be part of the same groups and amplify some of your responses.

While that means good information can be forwarded quickly and help obtained, it also raises the possibility that fake news or unnecessary messages that are anxiety-provoking (cue COVID-19 scares/cures) can also be spread equally fast. This is because, in each group, there will be many people who are present in multiple groups.

In the brain, these overlapping neurons within multiple neurotags serve firstly a protective response. More inputs that occur from multiple neuronal networks increase your chance for survival because of the better communicative capacity. Each neuron can be connected to almost millions of other neurons (imagine Taylor Swift and her Twitter followers).

Another advantage of multiple overlapping networks is a distribution of memory. For example, think about someone you love (your grandma, for instance). You will reflexively recollect her smell, the taste of some food that she would have prepared and you may often get a vivid recollection of a certain comment or language that she used. Alternatively, you may have a song from your childhood that on hearing will trigger certain associated memories, and these can then be powerful enough to bring about other changes in your body.

Neurotags and the networks are often involved in pain because they can interpret any damage to the body or possibly even impending damage as danger. If a preprogrammed network is present then spreading the message to protect against danger is much faster. This would be similar to you wanting to spread some information via Twitter – it is much easier for a message to go viral if you have a huge number of followers already. If you are just starting out then it takes time.

This concept of neural networks has now been identified for all sensations that we feel, such as anxiety, depression, suffering, anger, fear and disgust. If we have an experience that makes us feel many such emotions at the same time, for example a food poisoning episode that causes us to have nausea, vomiting, disgust, stomach pain and bloating, then all of this will fire off certain neurons in the brain that will then form a neural network. The next time you go to that same restaurant or get a whiff of that smell, it might cause you to experience those same emotions and induce a sensation of nausea as an early protection.

Because these networks have fired together, they will start to wire together. This is called Hebb's Law. The effect of this repeated firing and wiring is that you could have a sensation or emotion that causes a certain network to activate, but if this is overlapping with a 'pain' network then it will also worsen the pain.

Think of a time when you had a flare-up of your back/neck/knee pain. It doesn't mean that there has to be a structural problem with your disc or joint in your back or your cartilage in your knee every time you have a flare-up or that it gets inflamed every day. It is more likely – and indeed research has shown – that it is related to this principle of firing and wiring. It is more software-related and associated with the phenomenon of nerves that wire together, fire together.

It does also present hope and opportunity that if you can get your neurons firing in a different, positive way then you could potentially wire them together in a different network that can work to dampen pain.

The New Neuromatrix

A consequence of understanding the presence of neurotags and neural networks has meant that we have to redefine our understanding of what a pain pathway is. The presence of neural networks essentially means that pain is felt everywhere in the brain rather than in specific areas.

New Zealand-based public health and pain science researcher Elspeth Shipton conducted a study with her colleagues looking at 383 medical schools across many continents and noted disappointingly that 96 per cent of medical schools in the UK and USA and almost 80 per cent of European medical schools had no compulsory dedicated module on teaching about pain.[7] That matches up to how I

NERVE STRUCTURES THAT MEDIATE PAIN

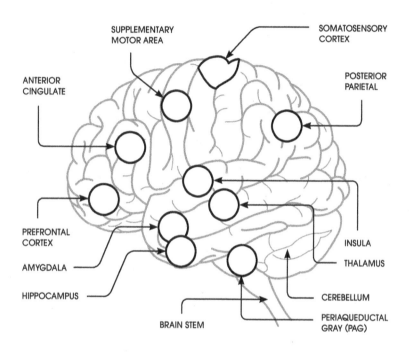

SUPPLEMENTARY MOTOR AREA

SOMATOSENSORY CORTEX

ANTERIOR CINGULATE

POSTERIOR PARIETAL

PREFRONTAL CORTEX

AMYGDALA

HIPPOCAMPUS

INSULA

THALAMUS

CEREBELLUM

BRAIN STEM

PERIAQUEDUCTAL GRAY (PAG)

was taught when I did my medical training in India, and I studied at a tertiary national institute.

In fact, as late as 2007, we were still taught that once we felt 'pain' signals in some part of the body, it would follow predetermined 'pain' nerves and these would reach up to a common gate at the base of the brain (thalamus). From there, the information would go to a specific motor or sensory centre, which would then determine how we move away from the 'pain'-causing stimulus.

At best, this is oversimplification and, at worst, it's just plain wrong. Even the father of the original trailblazing 'gate control theory', Patrick Wall, confessed, 'The labelling of nociceptors as pain fibres was not an admirable simplification, but an unfortunate trivialisation under the guise of simplification.'[8]

We now know that there are no 'pain nerves', nor are there specific 'pain' pathways. The nociceptive signals that come from a peripheral area travel via nerves and, when they reach the brain, they reach multiple points, collectively called the 'neuromatrix'.

These multiple structures of the matrix where the sensation of 'pain' integrates form neural networks. At this time, the main structures are thought to be the dorsal posterior insula, the prefrontal cortex, the hippocampus and the amygdala, but neurons that receive such signals and interpret them are present in every part of the brain.

Take for example the amygdala. We now know that the amygdala normally processes the sensations of emotion, memory, pleasure, sight, smell, fear and also pain. So if the sensation of pain were to arrive at the amygdala it would not just provoke the 'pain' network but it would also provoke feelings of anxiety and fear.

This is sometimes challenging to accept, but I see this in a lot of my patients – if you are extremely anxious about something else or are undergoing other stressors that bring on fear, then it will amplify your pain in an area of the body. If you did a scan on that area, it would look no different, but the intensity of pain for you is very real!

Looking at the table below, you can see the main areas of the brain in which the emotion of pain is perceived. You'll also notice that those areas have neurotags for other emotions and activities, which all get impaired when one has ongoing pain. Now think about why your pain feels much worse when you are more anxious, depressed or angry. Maybe you think of a traumatic time or see something on the TV/your phone that triggers a visual image in your brain that activates your pain area as well. So many patients tell me that they cannot recollect why their pain flared up suddenly when they were sitting on their sofa or watching TV.

Neural networks[9]

Area of the brain	Neural networks fire and wire for
Amygdala	Pain, emotion, memory, pleasure, sight, smell, emotional extremes
Hippocampus	Stores pain memories
Anterior cingulate	Pain, emotional self-control, sympathetic control, problem-solving
Orbital frontal cortex	Pain, understanding, emotional attachment, pleasant vs unpleasant evaluation
Somatosensory 1 and 2	Pain, touch, temperature, pressure, position, vibration
Prefrontal area	Pain, executive function, creativity, empathy, intuition
Posterior parietal lobe	Pain, sensory, visual and auditory perception, mirror neurons
Supplementary motor area	Pain and mirror neurons
Insula	Pain, temperature, itch, empathy, sensual touch, disgust, mirror neurons, amygdala control

Neural networks and predictive processing

Often before you experience pain, there is a lot of influence from your perception and your emotions, your thoughts and, more importantly, the context or the environment in which you are working or living. With chronic pain, all of this can amplify or dampen the signal, as we saw in the construction worker examples on pages 110–11. If your thoughts are extreme and negative because you do not know what is going to happen next, this will influence your final description of pain.

Neural networks and tags have now been combined with a newer understanding of the brain and how it is connected together. The 'bottom-up' model works by collecting information about the outside world with the help of nerve endings in the eyes, ears, skin and our intestine and muscles. This information is then sent via the nerves to the brain and the brain then interprets its meaning and creates a plan of action about the cause. This is the conventional way to look at pain so we expect to get the best benefit from surgeries or steroid injections, and it is the model on which the present biomedical way of healthcare is designed.

What it does not take into account is any possible top-down factors that could affect the perception, such as past experience or expectations. Predictive coding fills that gap.[10] In this model, the brain constantly keeps changing and adding to its perceptions and representations – if the perception is considered unfamiliar or dangerous, then the response changes accordingly. Expectation makes a big difference in deciding what the output of the prediction should be. This model is able to explain how expectation can influence our perception, unlike the bottom-up approach.

The high levels of the nervous system, which are effectively the uppermost parts of the brain, are constantly predicting what the sensations could be that could come to them. These predictions create a certain amount of nerve activity that flows down and meets any incoming signals from whatever has been happening.

When the two signals meet, a comparison is often made between what has been predicted and what arrives and, if it is close enough, then nothing changes and the world is seen as we expect it to be. However, if the error is quite big then the opportunity arises for the brain to update its model and remember it for the next time. So, how does this work for pain?

This understanding explains how past experiences, thoughts, actions, expectations and even emotions can all amplify the pain that one has, and sometimes this includes the very perception of pain itself.

Let's look at an example. I have been seeing Robert for the last few years. He has persistent low back pain and has had trials of injections that didn't work. Scans did not show anything that needed surgery. He hasn't been able to work for the last four years. His worst problem is bending backwards. As he confessed when I tried to encourage him to bend backwards as I was examining him, 'I do not want to, Doc. I think it might just go and I don't want to try and risk it.'

I realised that Robert's brain networks over time had now formed a prediction that every time he leans backwards, it would be painful. This introduces a strong bias for him. He thinks that if he leans back, it will soon mean that the nervous system starts producing the pain as a protective stimulus to prevent him doing any more.

It is therefore very important to understand and influence the top-down factors that are contributing to your pain experience; if you can, with support, try to do the movement you are hesitant to do, and you get no worsening of pain, it creates an error in your predictions. The brain can then update itself to the new model and, if that means doing some previously fearful movements, then that will be, in effect, a reduction in pain with better function. (See page 236 for more on this.)

HOW THE MIND THINKS

Professor of Psychiatry Steve Peters simplifies the complex working of the brain and mind into three parts:[11]

1. You, the human (capable of being rational and thinking logically).
2. A computer (that stores and retains memories of every experience you have had, whether you remember it or not).
3. A chimp or reptilian (which can function on its own, interprets events differently from you and is often very emotional and irrational and driven to protect you from anything it considers harmful).

The human part of the mind takes a long time to mature and can eventually control the computer and chimp/reptile, but the reptilian part of the brain is extremely fast and protective in nature. It is often hardwired into our bodies and is present from birth.

We can learn to influence the reptilian part and we can use the computer to help change it around, but this takes time. The reptilian and computer parts of the mind together form a machine and its primary responsibility is to react quickly to any danger in the environment and keep you safe.

When it overreacts, one of the ways it can present is pain. When we look at the influence of chronic stress in pain conditions like fibromyalgia, we can appreciate why the machine can tend to persistently overreact, especially when the stressor occurs earlier in life (see below). Appreciating the role of the stressor and how it affects the body gives us more management and treatment strategies.

The Mind–Body Connection

Due to the inherent nature of the biopsychosocial model of pain (see page 108) and the multiple neural networks shown above, it becomes clear that the mind and body are not separated, but instead share a deep connection with each influencing the other.

The false separation of mind and body does not help in the management and treatment of a complex condition like pain. The influence of chronic traumatic stress on the functioning of the brain and nervous system results in physical changes in various body systems, and these change the system, causing it to become more sensitive, overprotective and maladaptive.

The pervasive pain in conditions like fibromyalgia or widespread osteoarthritis starts to act like a chronic stressor and this means that the flight-fight-freeze response is constantly on alert. This causes exhaustion at multiple levels and results in accelerated 'wear and tear' on the multiple systems of the body – the hormonal, immune and nervous systems.

Chronic traumatic stress and adversity

When looking at chronic stress it's so important to appreciate the social element and the role that Adverse Childhood Experiences (ACEs) and developmental trauma play in the moulding of the neural networks and the immune system.

Research shows that if a person has been exposed to significant stress on the immune or nervous system as a child or teenager then there is a much higher risk of developing chronic pain and other long-term conditions such as diabetes and asthma. Many organisations working with pain/trauma patients now realise that trauma is very widespread and are

OVERARCHING EFFECT OF ADVERSITY

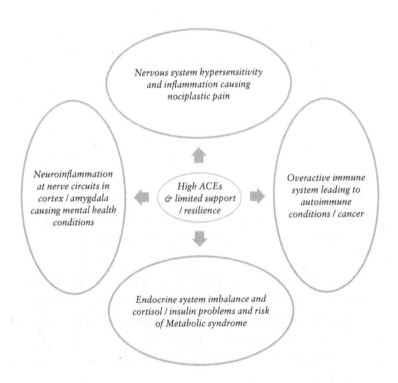

Nervous system hypersensitivity and inflammation causing nociplastic pain

Neuroinflammation at nerve circuits in cortex / amygdala causing mental health conditions

High ACEs & limited support / resilience

Overactive immune system leading to autoimmune conditions / cancer

Endocrine system imbalance and cortisol / insulin problems and risk of Metabolic syndrome

changing their way of understanding this by recognising trauma, responding to it in a compassionate manner and trying to avoid making it worse for pain patients. This is called a 'trauma-informed approach'.

The original ACE study explored Big Trauma (T), such as physical, sexual and emotional abuse, neglect and family dysfunction, and irrespective of which country this was done in, if people had experienced four or more such experiences, they had a significant increase in chronic pain and other diseases, including obesity, hypertension, cardiovascular disease, osteoarthritis and autoimmune conditions.[12]

Adult victims of childhood maltreatment report more intense chronic pain, headaches, abdominal and respiratory symptoms, gynaecological and neurological problems.[13] When people also then go on to experience relatively 'Small' Trauma (t) like bullying, #metoo, the stress of looking after children who may have health issues (ASD, ADHD, etc.) themselves, road traffic accidents, litigation, poverty, work stress and other social problems, rates of chronic pain will increase.

In the case of Debbie (who we met on page 105), she had nine out of the ten adverse experiences during her childhood, *plus* she was a single mother with two children who had ongoing mental health problems. Think about the combination of 't' and 'T' in her. Could that be a more unifying reason for her pain than all the multiple body parts that surgeons kept trying to operate on thinking that they were the pain generators?

We know that almost 50 per cent of the population might have experienced a major trauma and often the support you have from your family and friends/community can give you the resilience you need to overcome such adversity and thrive.

While the table below may not apply to many of you, it is worth exploring in order to understand yourself better and decide whether you want to seek professional help. If you have answered 'Yes' to four or more of these then your system is going to be just a little more vulnerable.

While you were growing up, during your first 18 years of life:	Yes	No
1 Did a parent or other adult in the household often or very often act in a way that made you afraid or emotionally abuse you?		
2 Did a parent or other adult in the household often or very often push, grab or hit you so hard that you had marks or were injured?		
3 Did an adult or person at least five years older than you ever attempt or actually sexually abuse you?		
4 Did you often or very often feel that no one in your family loved you or thought you were important or special?		
5 Did you often or very often feel that you didn't have enough to eat, had to wear dirty clothes and had no one to protect you? Or your parents were too drunk or high to take care of you or take you to the doctor if you needed it?		
6 Were your parents ever separated or divorced?		
7 Was your mother or stepmother often or very often slapped, kicked, hit with a fist or threatened with a gun or knife?		

8	Did you live with anyone who was a problem drinker or alcoholic or who used street drugs?		
9	Was a household member depressed or mentally ill, or did a household member attempt suicide?		
10	Did a household member go to prison?		

Mirror neurons

Literally called 'the neurons that shaped civilisation', mirror neurons discovered in the nineties provided a new way by which we understand how people imitate the actions of each other and how humans respond and generate empathy and sympathy, and even the evolution of language.[14] An example in the world of pain is if you see someone else suffering or wincing in pain, there is a good chance that your mirror neurons will be activated, thus allowing you to empathise and feel their pain. Mirror neurons have now been postulated to be present in many parts of the brain.

Mirror neurons explain why some therapies for certain pain conditions, like phantom limb pain or CRPS, would work. The use of mirror therapy may work because mirror neurons often get activated when you perform a certain task. They also get activated if you simply watch an action that you can do yourself, so they won't be activated if you see a bird flying, but they will be activated when you imagine or visualise an action that you're not even performing. This is apparently the reason why athletes often use visualisation of their race or sport so that they imagine the whole process many times in their head. By doing this, they are using the mirror neurons and setting up a new network (the principle of neuroplasticity) to drive and create new circuits.

Reframing belief and expectation

You may be wondering what the concept of reframing has to do with pain. Australian pain researcher Tasha Stanton carried out a series of studies in patients with low back pain, neck and knee pain (due to osteoarthritis).[15] Using visual illusions/video goggles and creaking noises when doing spine bending around the neck or back or stretching the knee, she showed that the brain combines different information from the eyes and ears to create a perception of increased pain. For example, in the back pain study, she was able to show that patients' feelings of how stiff their back was did not correlate with an objective measure of back stiffness.[16] So their perception was altered.

We'll explore this further in the next chapter, but I present this here to demonstrate the power of the mind–body connection. As the above example demonstrates, it is possible that our feeling of stiffness may be more in line with what we believe we are seeing or hearing rather than the actual muscle stiffness – it has a lot to do with how pain is perceived (our beliefs) and interpreted (reframed) by our nerves. That is a sobering thought on the power of our nervous system. In the same way, we might be willing to accept some kinds of pain/procedures if we are told beforehand that they will have a more beneficial intention to what we otherwise thought. This can be used to reduce the nocebo response or enhance the placebo response (see pages 78 and 76).

Social and physical pain

There is a substantial overlap between the nerve circuits that make sense of the signals of physical nociception and social pain. This was shown in a study where participants were asked to take part in a virtual ball-tossing game with a computer (Cyberball).[17] After some time in the second round, they got excluded from the game. All this while, their brains were being scanned in real time to see what regions were affected most. There was evidence of increased activity in the exact same areas of the brain where they would have felt physical pain. So rejection and loneliness can be as intense and disturbing as physical pain itself.

These similarities between social pain and physical pain show that if social factors, such as support, resilience and family and friend networks, are not adequate, then that in itself increases the vulnerability to chronic pain. Because of increased exposure to these major life stresses, this kind of vulnerability can result in an increased sensitivity to pain. If you find yourself in such a situation, it is not uncommon to find that you end up taking on unhealthy or maladaptive coping techniques, like drinking alcohol, eating sugary food/drinks or even taking drugs, thus putting you at risk of many other long-term conditions. Isolation, prolonged conflict and ostracism or stigmatisation due to a variety of reasons (racism or other minority ethnic issues, for example) can all cause social 'pain' and, since the systems overlap, these can amplify other bodily areas of pain.

If what I have said above resonates with you, try to reach out proactively to expand your social network. This may be local community or library-based activities. Choosing something that you find enjoyable to do along with someone else can help significantly in improving your health, both physically and mentally, and that will in turn reduce your pain. Involving your family members in such an activity can further reduce pain and improve belonging.

The Vagus Nerve

The vagus nerve is the tenth of the twelve cranial nerves that we have in our body. It is the longest nerve of the autonomic nervous system. With its wandering nature, we now understand that it is the supercharged two-way eight-lane highway that connects your brain to the rest of the body, carrying information to and fro between these structures. It has intricate links to the heart, the digestive tract and intestine, and finally to the immune system.

The gut–brain axis refers to the deep connection between the brain and the central nervous system to the intestinal nervous system (also called the second, or 'gut', brain). The vagus is the main nerve linking both these brains together.

Good bacteria in the gut influence the nervous and immune system and that information travels up through the vagus to bring about changes in the brain that can reduce anxiety and maintain mood. For example, the information and certain chemicals travel through the vagus to the hypothalamus and the limbic system. This is the part that influences and controls your emotions, so think about those 'gut' feelings and the 'butterflies in the tummy' that you get when you feel nervous.[18]

The vagus nerve represents an important junction and connection between various neurological, inflammatory and psychiatric diseases. Since it is a nerve, treatments for trying to influence the nerve have involved stimulating it using electricity or nutritional supplements and, in many cases, relaxation techniques like yoga and meditation. In all these techniques, the main aim is to use the vagus to influence how the main brain or second brain changes the production of chemicals, transmitters or hormones to reduce symptoms of pain and distress.

Polyvagal theory

This is a neurobiological construct introduced by professor of psychiatry and neuroscience researcher Stephen Porges in 1994.[19] He proposed, based on animal experiments, that the vagus has two branches: an older branch called the dorsal vagus nerve (which looks after the function of the intestine and lower limbs) and a newer branch called the ventral vagus nerve (which looks after the facial muscles and heart).

Within polyvagal theory, normal is when the newer branch of the vagus (ventral nerve) is active and we are social, engaged and happy. When we get aroused due to actual or perceived danger then we would activate the sympathetic nervous system (fight or flight response) to protect us. However, if the danger is too much and the chance of safety is very little, then the dorsal branch of the vagus kicks in, leading to a low arousal state and, at its extreme, a freeze or fall response, where we become immobilised or actually faint or dissociate.

If you are in pain for a long time and there is associated stress, trauma/anxiety or depression for any reason, then it is likely that you may be in a system dominated by the sympathetic or the dorsal vagus. Once the fight or flight reactions occur, it takes much longer for the body to come back into the pre-fight or flight state. Moving from those states to normal can be achieved through many ways, but it first requires us to have a sense of safety.

When you are in prolonged chronic pain or traumatic stress, activation of the dorsal branch can explain why you might have stomach problems diagnosed as IBS or pelvic pain, or even low back pain, when MRI scans do not show anything.

Often the three systems (the sympathetic, dorsal and ventral vagus) are in dynamic balance allowing for quick adjustments and fine-tuning. It is a very different way to understand the nervous system and, in some ways, it is again an oversimplification, but within pain and associated chronic emotional trauma it is quite useful in being able to offer many new therapies to people in pain.

A number of trauma-based therapists and psychologists are using these principles alongside cognitive behavioural therapy (CBT) to help pain patients where there is an overlap of mental health issues, like previous trauma, anxiety, depression or post-traumatic stress disorder (PTSD). If patients have had an unresolved childhood trauma or a significantly life-threatening/ongoing stressful event (such as an illness or care of a disabled partner/parent/sibling/child), then it changes the body's response to the trauma. This might mean using techniques like grounding and breathing to start with (see Chapter 9) and, when combined with some physical activity, it helps in releasing the chemicals and bringing the body back to the normal state.

The Brain's Dr Jekyll and Mr Hyde: Microglia[20]

The neuromatrix, or the neuronal theory, does not fully capture the complexity of chronic pain. For a long time, the brain has been thought of as not having an immune system, or at least not being affected by the body's immune problems. We now know that this is not true and that microglia – one of the three types of glial cells in the brain – are quite intimately involved with maintaining persisting pain.

Microglia constitute about 10 per cent of the total number of cells. They are self-renewing, long-lasting cells.[21] Long thought of as simple housekeepers and waste collectors, they are now understood to be representatives of the immune system in the brain. They share a common ancestor with the rest of the body's immune cells and around the eighth day of an embryo make their way up into the brain before the blood–brain barrier forms on the thirteenth day.

In their Dr Jekyll role (called M2), they nourish the neurons, kill them off when not needed and keep tabs on their overall number, health and function. In addition to the neurons, they also monitor the synapses – the junctions between two neurons where all the action happens. Microglia, along with another glial cell called astrocytes, help the synapses mature and form, model and sculpt them, and prune them when not needed.

Their Mr Hyde role (called M1) comes along when there is injury or stress, either acute or chronic. When this happens, they get activated and spew out inflammatory chemicals in the brain and spinal cord that can cause collateral damage to the neighbouring neurons and synapses and encourage astrocytes to amplify the damage. This kind of inflammation within the nervous system does not often present in the bloodstream and cannot be picked up yet with routine blood tests or scans. Drugs like opioids increase microglial activation.

It is now thought that gliopathy (a dysregulation of the microglia/astrocytes) is the main issue in chronic pain and central sensitisation, and our focus should be on preventing or modifying the action of Mr Hyde (microglial overactivation) and pushing it back to a Dr Jekyll state.

Many drugs are being studied that could modify the actions of microglia. These include minocycline, propentophyline, low dose naltrexone (LDN), cannabinoids (as microglia have cannabis receptors), immune therapies, metformin and mesenchymal stem cells.

What is also now understood is that the gut microbiome – the collective genes from our gut bacteria and organisms (more on this in Chapter 6) – regulates and shapes the function of the microglia. They send their signal via the vagus nerve to the brain and this can cause further chemicals to be released to activate or dampen the microglial function. Omega-3 fatty acids are shown to enhance the anti-inflammatory action. Bioactive compounds present in Mediterranean diets, like carotenoids and phenolic compounds, are also protective. Fasting diets and ketogenic diets also suppress activation of microglia. They all help in releasing healing mediators called resolvins, maresins and protectins to facilitate this.

Reduced signalling and production of the inflammation-related genes have been seen with mind–body therapies, specifically tai chi, qi gong, yoga and mindfulness meditation (see Chapter 9). Popular science journalist and award-winning author Donna Jackson Nakazawa highlights the benefits of magnetic stimulation (see page 296), EEG-based neurofeedback techniques and a fasting mimicking diet (similar to intermittent fasting and time-restricted diet – see page 179) as other non-drug approaches to dampening microglia activation and promoting health and well-being.[22]

THE SURVEILLANCE CAMERA

Our immune cells come equipped with a camera (called the TLR4), which detects anything it considers foreign or dangerous and triggers and creates an associated molecular pattern (AMP), which it commits to memory.[23] Such molecular patterns can be caused by viruses (like coronavirus) and bacteria (pathogen AMP), injuries and surgery (damage AMP), antibiotics/food toxins/opioids (xenobiotic AMP), fear and anxiety (behaviour AMP) and wrong thoughts/beliefs (cognitive AMP). You can see, therefore, how seemingly unrelated things like food toxins and fear and beliefs, and even stress, can all trigger the immune system and thereby sensitise the nervous system. These can often contribute to worsening pain.

Stress Regulation

Our classic understanding of the stress response involves the HPA (hypothalamus–pituitary–adrenal) axis and the sympathetic nervous system releasing cortisol and adrenaline to deal with threats that can come from either inside the body or the external environment. While it aims to be protective in acute situations, chronic ongoing traumatic stress causes long-term problems with the endocrine and neuroimmune systems.

Both acute (being involved in an accident, major surgery, abuse, a fight with a boss/loved one) or chronic (looking after an unwell family member, dealing with chronic illness, childhood adversity, divorce, pandemics) stressors all cause raised inflammatory markers. Sometimes you can detect this in the bloodstream. More often, this causes an inflammatory response in the brain, which, as I mentioned on page 134, cannot be seen on a scan or picked up in the bloodstream as yet. Particularly chronic traumatic stress, like ACEs, can prime the microglia for activation and then often a minor stressor can push it to recreate a neural inflammation and full-blown microglia activation. This affects the neural synapses in these areas and, combined with persistent high cortisol levels, changes various nerve circuits in the brain leading to inflammation in the immune system of the brain and spinal cord and elevation of pain and mood disorders.

Reducing the pro-inflammatory chemicals can therefore contribute to stress and pain reduction. While there are some drugs available for this, a more holistic approach using the MINDSET principles in this book can aid in reducing these chemicals in the brain and body. Mind–body therapies like yoga, acupuncture, dietary changes and mindfulness practices can all lower the chemicals and microglial activation.[24] This would also explain the increasing popularity of Eastern practices like Ayurveda and traditional Chinese medicine, as they often incorporate lifestyle approaches alongside dietary modifications and specific herbs.

Stress-reduction techniques

Pain – and any other trauma you face in life – is a stressor, which causes changes in the nervous system and in the brain, and can worsen pain. Therefore, putting in place stress-reduction strategies is vital and more important than any medications or recreational equivalents, like alcohol, sugary foods or smoking, in reducing your pain.

Relaxation response: Noted cardiologist and Harvard mind–body professor Herbert Benson's 'relaxation response' (with practice and training) aims to achieve 'flow or a focused awareness' of ourselves by using a repeated word, phrase, breath or action, such as 'OM' in meditation.[25] The use of Christian rosaries and the Hindu 'japa mala' are a form of focus on an object. One can use something as simple as counting one when taking in a breath and two when breathing out.

Breathing techniques: Techniques like 3–4–5 breathing (see page 280) or box breathing enable focused awareness. A stable breathing rhythm is the first step towards the relaxation response.

The 54321 technique: Once you have a good breathing technique to slow your heart rate down, the 54321 can be used to further reduce your stress and pain-induced anxiety. Look for five things you can see, four things you can touch, three things you can hear, two things you can smell and one thing you can taste. This forces you to use all your senses and can help dampen some of the pain.

Mindfulness practice: Adopting a passive non-judgemental attitude to your thoughts is core to mindfulness-based stress reduction (MBSR). There are a number of online apps and websites that allow you to try out these techniques (see Resources, page 310).

TOP TIPS FOR STRESS REDUCTION

- Gentle **exercise**: start small, for short durations and then build up.
- **Enforce** relaxation by body scans, progressive relaxation exercises, guided imagery.
- **Expect** the unexpected: write a plan for what you will do.
- **Embrace** positive experiences and do something you love.
- **Encourage** the mind to think positively.
- **Enable** yourself to say NO when needed for self-care.
- **Engage** your network to socialise and reach out for help.

TOP TIPS FOR STRESS AVOIDANCE

- Planned rest.
- Regular routine.
- Learn to pace yourself.
- Create a supportive network.
- Understand and know your stressors – what sets you off, be it people, foods or situations.

I hope you now understand the powerful influence your nervous and immune systems can have in amplifying both pain and stress. Understanding this complex relationship itself can be very helpful and often sets the stage for patients to manage and lower their stress, and thus reduce a big contributor to their worsening pain.

This chapter has hopefully given you some ways to understand your pain and recognise and manage stress. The next chapter will give you a safe and evidence-based method to further reduce your stress and pain. An important way to calm your immune and nervous systems is to calm your second brain (the gut) using nutrition, so let's now look at the role diet can play in overcoming pain.

Summary

- The nervous system and its interaction with the immune system of the brain can maintain chronic pain.
- The brain and the nervous system function like a predictive machine to protect you.
- Pain is an alarm system that can often become faulty in its wiring.
- Pain is modified throughout the nervous system and can be affected by diet, context and environment.
- Microglia can cause low-grade inflammation in the brain and can activate stress.
- A number of non-drug techniques aimed at stress modification and diet can all reduce inflammation in the brain and body, easing pain.

CHAPTER 6

Diet and the Microbiome

What happens in the vagus, doesn't just stay in vagus.
Professor John Cryan, neuroscientist and researcher

MANY OF MY patients are quite surprised when I ask them about their dietary habits when they come for a consultation. A few years ago, it wasn't even part of my practice. However, increasingly, I have become more aware of the problems of our present-day diets. Everywhere I looked, lifestyle and diets were being explored for obesity control, diabetes and blood pressure management. I wondered whether they could also have a role in pain, especially if there was no nociception.

After I completed a course on nutrition and chronic pain, I was amazed to discover that when there is neuroinflammation – inflammation in the immune system of the brain and spinal cord – nutritional techniques seemed to be more effective than drugs in some cases and are beneficial without any obvious side effects. Scientific evidence now shows that good nutrition protects against excessive inflammation in various parts of the body.

I learnt that, if nociception is present, nutrition can be combined with medications and interventions to enhance their benefit. If there was no nociception yet people had pain, nutrition had a much better chance of making a meaningful difference than any drug.

If there was nociplastic pain (central sensitisation – see page 53), especially in conditions like fibromyalgia where people have significant fatigue/widespread pain and 70 per cent have IBS, then nutrition and diet changes can also help.

In many autoimmune disorders, like rheumatoid arthritis and lupus where nociplastic or mixed pain is present in more than 25 per cent of patients, nutrition could present a valuable way of managing symptoms without side effects.

The phenomenon of central sensitisation is known to be present in many other chronic pain conditions, like osteoarthritis, migraine headaches and IBS, and dietary interventions can result in significant improvements for many sufferers with very few side effects.

This came home to me in a dramatic fashion with Sarah.

Sarah's story

Sarah was referred to me by her rheumatologist for further management of her pain and fatigue. She had a diagnosis of secondary fibromyalgia alongside rheumatoid and psoriatic arthritis, both of which were under remission on strong drugs that modified the immune system. She was in her early forties but looked considerably older and tired. Though she had been diagnosed with the rheumatology conditions about three years ago, she had symptoms she had felt for almost a decade. Her immune system had affected a wide variety of her body's tissues and organs.

Despite the fatigue and multiple medications, which included a few pain medications along with methotrexate and hydroxychloroquine, Sarah was mum to two teenagers and tried to lead a relatively normal life. Apart from the pain and fatigue, she suffered from headaches, IBS and depression. Her GP had started her on antidepressant medications and her gastroenterologist had given her some IBS-related pills. Like so many other patients with autoimmune conditions referred to me, I wasn't sure what else I could do beyond increasing her pain medications and offering stronger drugs.

During the next six months, Sarah had two flare-ups of the fibromyalgia and each time she had her dosage increased, her symptoms got worse and she now complained of worsening IBS and chest and joint pain, and worsening 'fibro fog'/forgetfulness. She ended up being prescribed a course of high-dose oral steroids to help with the flare, but that had its own side effects.

Sarah's diet was significantly impacted and, not surprisingly, she was resorting to more processed food and takeaways as she was too fatigued to care for herself or for her family. I sent her to the dietician I work with who practises a functional and lifestyle medicine approach to health. Over the next six months, Sarah was advised and supported to make some changes in her diet. Although she found this initially difficult, she wanted to make the changes for her family's sake. She had had enough of all the side effects with the drugs and there were no further options anyway.

When I saw her in my follow-up, I was so surprised and delighted by the cheerier and happier Sarah sitting in front of me. She was a changed person, with obvious weight loss and in a much better mood than I had ever seen. When I asked her what had made the difference, she said an important factor was the support of her family, good coaching and a plan from the dietician. The recommendations that she followed enabled her to get a significant improvement in fatigue with better sleep and reduced pain and medication.

In this chapter, you will understand how you, too, can influence and modify/reduce, and in some cases even eliminate, your pain by looking more carefully at what you eat. Hopefully by the end of this chapter, you will understand:

- How chronic (persistent) pain is affected by the intestinal microbes and their genes.
- How eating some foods can cause inflammation in the gut, which can spread to the immune system of the brain and spinal cord.
- Whether you are eating a diet that puts you at risk.
- How being obese in itself can cause pain.
- That aiming for an anti-inflammatory diet will give you a safe and effective weapon against chronic pain.

Chronic Pain and the Microbiome

One of the features of the modern world that we live in is that infectious diseases – like COVID-19 – are generally rare. Waterborne diseases are also rare due to good public health measures like sanitation and hygienic practices. Social distancing measures and hand hygiene have also helped, especially in the developed world.

If you look more closely, however, autoimmune conditions like rheumatoid arthritis, type 1 diabetes, allergies to various substances, obesity, digestive problems and mental health conditions are all on the rise. Even chronic pain is at epidemic levels.

Linking all these vastly different medical conditions is a common thread. Scientists are convinced that the microbiome – the genes of the microbes that we collaborate and evolved with – has been affected and that it may have a major role to play in the rise of these so-called twenty-first-century diseases. This has now been shown with major research projects like the Human Microbiome Project.

There are about 100 trillion microbes (give or take a few trillion depending on which book or paper you read) that live in and on us. They are mostly bacteria, but there are other organisms like viruses, fungi and archaea that collectively are called the microbiota. When you include the genes from all of these organisms, there are roughly 4.4 million genes, which collectively are called the microbiome.[1]

The microbiome combines and collaborates with our 21,000–23,000 human genes to form a superorganism that helps us survive and thrive in this world. It is what makes us superior to the rice plant, which has circa 46,000 genes, and the water flea, which has approximately 31,000 genes.

The microbiota that live within us and alongside us help us digest the foods that we eat. Not only that, they digest food that we can't handle by ourselves, like some forms of fibre. They also process and detoxify many of the dangerous chemicals that we eat. Most importantly, they train and regulate the immune and nervous system of the intestine (the second brain) and, indirectly, the body and the first brain via the vagus and microglia cells (see pages 132 and 134). Not surprisingly, they also prevent the growth of more dangerous bacteria when they are looked after.

However, our modern lifestyle is causing the normal diversity of the microbiome to be lost/disturbed. Science writer and evolutionary biologist Alanna Collen identifies two very evident themes due to this disturbance or loss of the healthy microbes in her book, *10% Human*:[2]

1. The disturbance of the immune system lining the intestine that causes it to start fighting against its own. It is now possible that a number of pain conditions like fibromyalgia are also thought to have some level of autoimmune-related inflammation.
2. The dysfunction or abnormal function of the gut/intestine. Now you can look at the start of IBS from a different perspective.

Human immune cells are found in greater numbers in the gut than anywhere else in the body – 60–80 per cent of our immune system is in our intestines. Our intestinal wall is just one cell thick. This means that there is just one tiny layer between the blood and the 'outside world', so it makes sense to mobilise the body's defence forces where they are needed most and to have the maximum security and surveillance in this area.

This activation of the defence forces can mean that they can release potent chemicals to protect the body from the unhealthy or bad microbes. In the process, if some of those chemicals enter our bloodstream they can contribute to fatigue and central sensitisation (see page 53).[3]

CENTRAL SENSITISATION FROM GUT

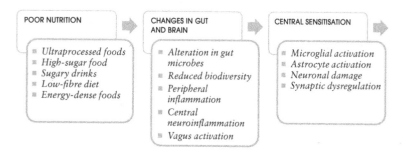

POOR NUTRITION	CHANGES IN GUT AND BRAIN	CENTRAL SENSITISATION
▪ Ultraprocessed foods ▪ High-sugar food ▪ Sugary drinks ▪ Low-fibre diet ▪ Energy-dense foods	▪ Alteration in gut microbes ▪ Reduced biodiversity ▪ Peripheral inflammation ▪ Central neuroinflammation ▪ Vagus activation	▪ Microglial activation ▪ Astrocyte activation ▪ Neuronal damage ▪ Synaptic dysregulation

The mechanism of how central nervous system sensitisation happens because of poor nutrition can be visualised as follows:

If you generally have a poor diet (low in fibre and energy-dense, meaning lots of carbohydrates) with no long-term proteins, vitamins or nutrients (think of a burger and chips and, no, a sprig of lettuce doesn't count!), then you have a higher chance of inflammatory chemicals in your body produced as a result of that diet. There are more free radicals (harmful reactive atoms of oxygen) and this can cause cell and tissue damage throughout the body.

This activates receptors inside the body called TLRs (toll-like receptors). These are like the surveillance cameras on many cells in your body on the lookout for anything they consider foreign. Once the TLRs are activated, they trigger a sensitisation along with inflammation in the spinal cord and the brain. In the brain they cause an activation of the policemen within the brain, known as the glial cells.

The glial cell activation results in what we call 'neuroinflammation'. This kind of glial cell overactivity causes further release of inflammatory chemicals and this combination of inflammatory chemicals with glial activation is seen in patients with chronic low back pain, fibromyalgia and even sciatica-like symptoms.

This indicates that even if the problem might have started in a joint or structure, over time other aspects like poor nutrition can contribute to the brain becoming sensitised and therefore amplifying the pain.

The nervous system does require certain nutrients for effective function. If the diet does not provide these nutrients, especially certain vitamins, then these deficiencies can also cause pain. For example, vitamin B12 deficiency can cause peripheral nerve pain and vitamin D deficiency can cause widespread pain symptoms in multiple joints and bones of the body. Quite frankly, in a provocative manner, every disease begins in the gut!

Like the mind–body connection, which we explored in the previous chapter (page 125), the brain and the gut are related and connected not just by chemicals but also by the vagus nerve (see page 132). Information flows both ways, so the mind can control the gut and the gut can influence the mind.

Our immune system in the gut becomes the first security and defence system against outside invaders. The immune system has to develop a method to recognise and archive the familiar friendly neighbourhood microbes that we normally live with and that the body has to work with.[4] Once this is done, it can then recognise the invaders and mount an attack to protect the body. All of this information and memory is then shared with the brain, but is also stored within the second brain (the enteric/intestinal nervous system). This 'gut brain' ensures that most of the gut activity, like digestion, is carried on independently without us being aware, unless it is really necessary.

Many of the microbes live within the intestine attached to the thin wall and often just one layer of cells separates them from the immune cells of the gut, which means that there is a lot of 'small talk' that occurs between them and the immune cells. So when you are feeling stressed or in pain, or are feeling full after a meal or even hungry, the information transfer between your gut and brain is 'overheard' by the microbes and they can influence it for the better or worse. This has been shown to happen both in animal and human studies where emotional states can be affected or changed by the presence or absence of these microbes, which is why a lot of scientists now think of the gut–brain axis as the gut–microbiota–brain axis.

And it goes both ways: the gut and brain keep influencing each other.

How does the brain influence the gut?

As we saw in the previous chapter, the brain develops certain pre-prepared neural networks or programs. These are often quick, hardwired shortcuts that allow us to deal with fight or flight responses, or any other stressful situations, and are there to help us survive and thrive.[5]

These emotional or neural networks are most often developed in connection with fear, anger, sorrow, play, lust, love and maternal support. To a small extent, these are dependent on our genes, but they are heavily influenced by events that we experienced early in our life. Such events can often sensitise and prime the microglia to be ready to protect at a later date.

Because of the mind–body connection through the vagus nerve, our response to these stressors is mirrored in our gut by making it more sensitive and bringing about symptoms such as nausea, irritability, diarrhoea and cramps. When these events happen, they get tagged and can be expressed again as a quick-response program any time in the future when another stressor comes along. This is very useful if you are encountering life or death situations, but can be a liability if you are otherwise safe.

How does the gut influence the brain?

The function of our digestive system and intestines is not just to digest food. We now know that there are hormone-producing cells located within our intestine that are responsible for producing 90 per cent of our serotonin.[6] Serotonin is an important signalling molecule, not just for digestion – it also gets transported to the brain for such vital functions as pain sensitivity, sleep, appetite, mood and overall well-being. It also acts to regulate the function and development of the microglia (see page 134).

This transfer occurs through the thick cables of the vagus nerve. Mood disturbances and mental health conditions like anxiety and depression are exceedingly common in pain patients and it is possible that some of this may be driven by a combination of gut dysfunction that is making the immune and hormone systems abnormal.

This bidirectional nature of communication from the gut to the brain and back integrates the immune, nerve and hormone signals, which is why microbes are now considered to be fundamental in maintaining the balance between the systems. In chronic pain conditions like IBS, inflammatory bowel disease or fibromyalgia, dysregulation of this communication can actually worsen the pain.

It makes sense, therefore, that influencing the microbiome in a positive manner should change the intensity of pain.

What Inflames the Gut and Causes Pain?

Now you know that you are a superorganism who lives alongside your most friendly neighbours, it is important to know what the consequences can be when you fall out with them or don't treat them right! This state of falling out with the microbiota and the irregular function of the gut–brain axis is called 'dysbiosis' and is understood to be a fundamental problem in IBS and often a major issue in fibromyalgia, migraine, inflammatory bowel diseases (Crohn's), Ehlers-Danlos syndromes, osteoarthritis and even rheumatoid arthritis.

Poor-quality foods

Energy-dense, highly processed foods and high-sugar drinks that release sugar quickly or bad fats (takeaway foods) can all cause inflammation and reduce diversity.

Drugs (antibiotics/pain medications)

Antibiotics and many other drugs, including chemotherapy and immunotherapy drugs, can all wipe out entire microbial populations. Infectious diseases or any stomach bug do the same by releasing toxins that can again kill off healthy populations of microbes. There are a number of case reports and scientific literature documenting the onset of chronic fatigue, ME or fibromyalgia-like symptoms after an infection for which antibiotics have been given.

Low variety of foods

'Low biodiversity' is the consequence of our dietary choices. Our adoption of the SAD (standard American diet), which is characterised by high intakes of red processed meat, pre-packaged foods, fried foods, refined grains, corn (and high-fructose corn syrup) and high-carbohydrate drinks, contributes significantly to low biodiversity over time.

Low biodiversity is often seen either in young or old age and is also noted in mental health and neurological disorders. Low biodiversity is also seen in some patients who cannot tolerate or become allergic to a variety of foodstuffs. Some strict diets can also cause this low biodiversity and that can become a problem and promote inflammation because it may allow another kind of microbe to flourish instead.

Wrong place/wrong time

This is a slight variation where patients may have had either an antibiotic or an unusual stomach bug that wipes out a certain population of microbes. This can be followed by an overgrowth of the unwanted microbe in a different area of the intestine where it would not normally expect to be. This

LEAKY GUT

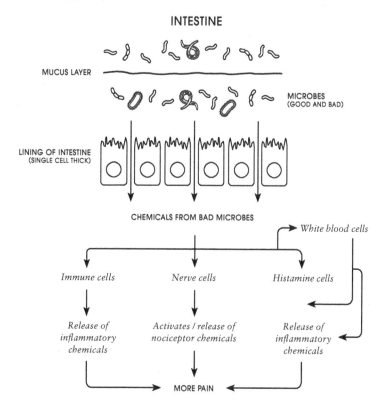

is seen in the condition of small intestinal bacterial overgrowth (SIBO), which is noticed very often in fibromyalgia and IBS patients. The body reacts with an inflammatory response affecting the normal function, causing pain, bloating, cramps and diarrhoea with nausea. It can be quite disabling and difficult to treat, and is thought to be due to the bad bacteria causing the lining of the single cell junction to swell and separate, causing a leaky gut.

Are You Living a Pro-Inflammatory Lifestyle?

Now that we've seen how chronic pain can be promoted, maintained and amplified by dysbiosis and low biodiversity, I hope you can see why paying attention to your diet and food and looking after your microbiome is vitally important because they can influence so many aspects of your physical and mental health. Introducing diversity and having a healthy gut seem to be essential to developing a normal inflammatory pain response.[7]

Mice can be bred in labs that have no microbes at all. They are called germ-free mice. When such mice are subjected to painful responses, there is reduced perception of pain to any inflammation.[8] This does not mean that pain can be reduced if you wipe out your microbes. Conversely, it shows that modifying the intestinal microbiome by giving various probiotics can alter the pain response. Another study in osteoarthritis showed that there is an association between the intensity of knee and hip pain and the kind of microbiomes that people have.[9]

Eminent gastroenterologist, author and neuroscientist Professor Emeran Mayer talks about a 'state of sub-optimal health', calling it a 'pre-disease' state.[10] I see several such patients in my clinic and a large number of chronic pain patients start out in that situation. They are often generally healthy, but due to a combination of life circumstances or work pressures and chronic pain, are often chronically stressed or tired. They have limited time and energy for daily exercise and self-care, and are borderline obese with poor dietary habits of fast food, packaged sandwiches and sugary drinks taken during short lunch breaks. They experience poor sleep, symptoms of fatigue and recurrent aches and pains, which sometimes get diagnosed as varying degenerative diseases if they present to their GP.

This prolonged stress system activation affects the gut–microbiota–brain axis and brings about a low-grade systemic inflammation in the body and neuroinflammation in the brain. Such inflammation can also occur within the gut, causing the release of more inflammatory chemicals called lipopolysaccharides (LPS), causing a leaky gut.

Gut reactions from chronic stressful situations and adversity either in childhood or adulthood don't just upregulate the pain we feel in our gut, but also in the rest of the body. Unfortunately, such stress levels end up reinforcing the need for more comfort foods – ultra-processed high-sugar foods – which only make things worse in terms of chronic pain.

Answer the questions below to see whether your present diet could be contributing to the inflammation levels in your body.[11]

		Yes	No
1	Do you have some form of processed takeaway food every day? Daily processed foods increase inflammation within the gut with no time for the body to heal itself.		

2	Do you have processed meat every day? Processed meat is high in saturated fat and releases a dangerous form of fats called trans fats, which are very inflammatory.		
3	Do you have refined flour/bread products every day (such as croissants/burger buns, etc.)? Refined bread products are digested far too quickly and promote overgrowth of bad bacteria.		
4	Do you have insufficient fibre in your diet? Fibre removes toxins from the gut, acting like a broom to sweep them out. Highly processed foods have very little fibre.		
5	Do you have insufficient phytonutrients in your diet daily? Phytonutrients are primarily found in fruits, vegetables, nuts and seeds, and have anti-inflammatory and antioxidant properties, which quench inflammation.		
6	Do you do insufficient exercise every day i.e. fewer than 30 minutes of moderate activity, such as walking, per day? Adipose tissue (fat) is pro-inflammatory.		
7	Do you think there is fatty acid imbalance in your diet? Trans fats lead to inflammation. This usually happens with more takeaway and processed foods consumed on a daily basis.		
8	Do you have issues with emotional stress and toxic relationships? They can promote inflammation, impair wound healing and promote immunosuppression.		

If you have answered yes to more than five of the questions above, then I would strongly recommend that you look to make a change to your dietary habits as they could well be contributing to your pain. The problem with a pro-inflammatory lifestyle is not just the fact that the foods can cause inflammation locally in the gut, but once they are stored in your body, they can release further inflammatory chemicals (adipokines) that can cause pain.

THE SOCIAL ASPECT OF FOOD

While this may seem an odd place to talk about this, I think the social aspects around eating play a very important role in our food habits and why and how we eat. Our context and whom we eat with can have powerful influences on how much we eat, what we eat and how it affects our mood.[12] Sometimes eating with family and friends in a social setting will keep us more accountable to sticking to healthier habits and certainly we will be influenced by them reciprocally.[13] Eating in isolation removes these advantages and can further worsen mental and physical health. While the work culture and working patterns of the modern generation have promoted eating alone, I think we must make a spirited attempt to eat at least one meal a day in a social setting with others.

Obesity and Pain

We all knew that obesity was a big risk for diabetes and other heart-related conditions. With COVID-19 we became aware that it was also possibly a high risk for catching the virus. As early as 2013, the Food and Agriculture Organization of the United Nations (FAO) announced that 25 per cent of Britons were obese and roughly 50 per cent of the UK population is projected to be obese by the year 2030.[14]

BODY MASS INDEX (BMI)

This is calculated by dividing your weight in kilograms by your height in metres squared. If your BMI is between 18.5 and 24.9 then you are in the healthy weight range. Between 25 and 29.9 is overweight, with more than 30 being classified as obese. Knowing your BMI is useful because it will give you a good idea of your starting point and whether there is a risk that obesity is influencing your pain.

Many people believe that pain is to be expected because being obese means that you are putting more pressure on the joints (leg/back/shoulders, etc.). However, that is only part of the story. We now understand that a more serious and deeper issue is going on.

There are various reasons for obesity to cause pain:

Mechanical loads

Obesity can increase the mechanical load on the spine, thus causing higher pressure forces. A survey of more than a million Americans showed that people with a BMI between 30 and 34 had 68 per cent more pain, but if their BMI was between 35 and 39 they had 136 per cent more pain.[15]

Researchers in Denmark did a postal survey of almost 29,000 twin subjects and noted that obesity was associated with low back pain and played a part in maintaining the chronic nature of the pain.[16] Australian researchers were able to show that osteoarthritis in the hip and knee was seven times higher in obese patients.[17]

Reduced blood flow

Obesity can put pressure on certain areas, causing reduced blood flow, thus increasing the risk of nerve damage (neuropathic pain).

Widespread inflammation

We now understand that people who are obese are likely to feel more pain due to a number of inflammatory chemicals in their bloodstream. The adipocyte (fat cell) itself releases inflammatory chemicals (cytokines) called IL-6 (interleukin 6), TNF alpha and leptin. This combination of chemicals ends up activating the nervous system, resulting in a bigger outpouring of cytokines and causing central sensitisation. Since a lot of the fat can be stored in and around the intestines (visceral fat), it can affect the local nervous and immune system, thus starting off a process in the brain. If you are obese and feeling pain then it may not be a nociceptive pain (i.e. from your joint arthritis getting worse) but actually a nociplastic pain because of the involvement of your brain and nerves. So it's important to think very carefully before going for injections or surgery just because of obesity.

Obesity is now considered a pro-inflammatory state that can increase cortisol (stress hormone), and this kind of chronic stress then ends up activating the neuroinflammation as well. This complicated relationship between being obese and having pain and inflammation can cause cells to become resistant to insulin, thus increasing the risk of getting diabetes and hypertension, and a more complex and dangerous set of conditions together called metabolic syndrome.

The Anti-Inflammatory Diet

Nutrition and dietary choices are often very personal and it can be quite difficult to get it right for everyone. However, when you are in pain and you have decided to embrace nutrition there are some top tips that will work with any diet:

- Look to eliminate pro-inflammatory foods in your diet.
- Add in anti-inflammatory foods – an anti-inflammatory diet is ideal for pain.
- Aim to drink 1–1.5 litres of water a day.
- Consider supplementing your diet with nutrients and vitamins/minerals.
- Consider eating all your food within an 8–12-hour window (try to leave time for your intestine to clean up in between).

Before we explore these further, let's first take a look at how healthy your diet currently is.

Healthy diet quiz[18]

Think carefully about the following questions and then circle your answers.

1. How much fruit do you normally eat each day (75g fresh or dried fruit, 1 medium piece, 250ml unsweetened juice)?

A. 0 (-2)
B. 1 (0)
C. 2–3 (+2)
D. 4 or more (+3)   (score) _____

2. How many vegetable servings do you normally eat each day (220g leafy greens, 100–110g any other veggie, raw or cooked)?

A. 0 (-4)
B. 1 (0)
C. 2 (+1)
D. 3 (+2)
E. 4 or more (+3)   (score) _____

3. How many different varieties of vegetables do you eat in a normal month?

A. 2 or less (-4)
B. 3–4 (0)
C. 5–6 (+1)
D. 7–8 (+3)
E. 9 or more (+4)   (score) _____

4. How many times do you eat dried beans or peas (legumes, lentils, chickpeas, kidney beans, green peas, etc.) in a normal week?

A. 0 (-2)
B. 1–2 (0)
C. 3–4 (+1)
D. 5–6 (+2)
E. 7 or more (+3)   (score) _____

5. How many times do you eat red meat in a normal week?

A. 6 or more (-4)
B. 4–5 (-3)
C. 1–3 (-1)
D. Less than once a week (+2)
E. 0 (+3)   (score) _____

6. How many times do you eat in a fast food restaurant in a normal week?

A. 6 or more (-5)
B. 4–5 (-4)
C. 1–3 (-3)
D. Less than once a week (-2)
E. 0 (0)   (score) _____

7. In a typical day, what do you drink most often?

A. Fizzy drinks (regular or diet) (-4)
B. Caffeinated coffee or tea (-1)
C. Decaffeinated coffee or tea (0)
D. Milk or fruit juice (0)
E. Herbal tea or water (+3)   (score) _____

8. How many 330ml cans of fizzy drink do you drink in a normal day?

A. 6 or more (-5)
B. 4–5 (-4)
C. 2–3 (-3)
D. 1 (-2)
E. Less than 1 (-1)
F. 0 (0)   (score) _____

9. How often do you eat fish in a typical week?

A. Never (-2)
B. Once (+1)
C. Twice (+2)
D. 3–5 times (+3)   (score) _____

10. In a typical week, how often do you eat whole grains (100 per cent wholegrain bread, whole oats, brown rice, quinoa, whole rye crackers)?

A. Never (-3)
B. 1–2 times a week (-1)
C. 3–4 times a week (0)
D. 5–6 times a week (+1)
E. 1 or more times a day (+3)   (score) _____

11. How often do you eat sweets such as biscuits, cakes or ice cream?

A. 1 or more times a day (-3)
B. Every other day (-2)
C. Twice a week (-1)
D. Once a week (0)
E. 2–3 times a month (+1)
F. Rarely (+3)   (score) _____

Your Total Score_____

Now add up your points (numbers in parentheses) and see how you scored:

22–28: Great eating habits
17–21: Pretty good eating habits
10–16: Needs some improvement
9 or less: Needs much improvement; try to change one habit at a time

Eliminating pro-inflammatory foods

Inflammatory carbohydrates

Carbohydrates are considered one of the three main food groups. Certain studies that were done in the sixties prompted a change to a low-fat, high-carbohydrate diet and, based on certain questionable concerns around cholesterol and fat, we have been taught that high fat can contribute to cardiovascular disease. We now know this isn't true. However, carbohydrates – especially the refined versions – have become universal. Most processed and refined carbohydrates (white bread and rice, pizza dough, many cereals, pastries, sugary desserts and pasta) are pro-inflammatory when consumed in excess, especially when the glycaemic index is high.

THE GLYCAEMIC INDEX (GI)

This is the measure of how carbohydrates influence blood sugar levels. It is measured on a scale of 0 to 100. Table sugar has a GI of 62. It is recommended that foods have a GI less than 55, which means they will be more slowly digested and metabolised, thus reducing inflammation. Foods higher than 65 are not recommended as they will contribute to inflammation, high sugar levels and spikes of insulin, which over time can be harmful. Consider swapping white rice with brown rice, instant oatmeal with steel cut oats, cornflakes with bran flakes, white potatoes with cauliflower mash, and white bread with wholegrain bread.

Since sugar itself is inflammatory (not to mention very addictive), another important aspect is the amount of extra sugar (or free sugars) that is added to foodstuffs. The recommendations are that no more than 5 per cent of our daily energy intake should come from these free sugars. That equates to 30g per day for adults and 24g for children. Assuming that 4g is roughly one teaspoon, that works out at an average of 7.5 teaspoons per day, and even lower for children.[19] The WHO now recommends that we aim to keep these free sugars to fewer than 6 teaspoons per day. To get a better sense of what that means, take a look at Dr David Unwin's sugar infographics at phcuk.org/sugar.[20]

To help you reduce your sugar intake, consider joining an organisation such as That Sugar Movement (see Resources, page 311).

> ### TOP TIP
>
> Aim to keep your sugar intake to fewer than 6–8 teaspoons a day. As a starter, calculate how much you are having in a day and try to reduce it by 10 per cent.

Inflammatory fats

After carbohydrates, eliminating bad fats is an ideal next step. Trans fats are by far the worst and come as natural and artificial. Artificial trans fatty acids occur when vegetable oils are chemically altered to stay solid in order to increase flavour and the shelf life of products. They can cause a significant rise in inflammation, especially when people are already obese. They are found in all processed foods (see box opposite).

It's important to note that not all fats are created bad. That old myth was due to poor interpretation of clinical studies and it is now accepted that cholesterol is essential for your brain function and health, and that dietary cholesterol does not really impact on your risk of heart disease.[21] However, cholesterol-rich foods have high quantities of saturated fatty acids like lauric acid, palmitic acid and myristic acid, which can increase levels of LDL (bad) cholesterol.[22] Examples of foods that are rich in such acids include: red meat and animal fat, butter, ice cream, lard and oils like palm kernel oil and coconut oil.

Omega-3 and omega-6 are two polyunsaturated fatty acids that are obtained from food. Omega-3 has more anti-inflammatory properties while omega-6 in high doses promotes inflammation. Before processed foods became the new normal, we ate similar quantities of omega-3 and omega-6. However, since our diet has changed from predominantly plant-based to a more high energy density, ultra-processed one, especially with an increase in the intake of sugars, this has changed the normal dietary balance between the omega-6 and omega-3 fatty acids. The amount of omega-6 has increased tremendously and the ratio is now around 15–25:1. This ratio is important because omega-6 potentially increases the amount of inflammatory chemicals in our body if taken in excess and that can cause or worsen pre-existing pain.

Try to completely remove trans fats/any ultra processed foods from your diet, and reduce your consumption of omega-6-rich food, such as vegetable oils, soybean oil, poultry and fast foods.

FOOD PROCESSING

Unprocessed

These foods have been picked straight from the orchard or farm and are usually in their natural state – fresh or frozen with minimal processing like cleaning or drying. Examples would include fresh and frozen fruit/vegetables/poultry/meat/seafood, eggs and egg whites, raw shelled nuts/seeds, intact whole grains and naturally fermented foods like miso, kimchi and sauerkraut/chutney.

Processed

These are extracted and then concentrated to extend their shelf life by milling, refining or hydrogenation. They are acceptable in small quantities, but do build up and can contribute to issues. Examples are butter, cheese, margarine, sugar, maple syrup, flour containing lactose and gluten, cream, corn syrup and dried fruits.

Ultra processed

These are often highly processed by baking, frying or deep frying and have additives, flavours and preservatives. They can trigger the brain reward centres and as such need to be eliminated if possible. Examples include bacon, white bread, biscuits, cakes, sweets, chips, doughnuts, ice cream, crisps, sausages and smoked/cured meats.

Allergens like gluten/lactose

The next food groups to consider reducing/eliminating are gluten and dairy products. Gluten refers to a couple of proteins (gliadin and glutenin) that are found extensively in wheat-based products, barley and rye. While its glue-like nature gives texture and consistency, gluten can activate the immune system in certain populations, causing intolerance and allergies. Similarly, dairy products contain lactose as their main carbohydrate. In some people who lack the enzyme to break down lactose, this causes an allergy and intolerance to dairy products. A number of studies have shown that lactose intolerance is quite prevalent and gluten allergies can also be present. The reasons for this are numerous and are beyond the scope of this book.

Sarah, who we met earlier, had an undiagnosed gluten allergy and one of the big reasons for her improvement was eliminating gluten from her diet. She realised that gluten and other heavier starches were not getting broken down effectively in the initial parts of her intestine. Some other microbes then break up gluten to release certain chemicals, which contributed to her leaky gut. This caused some chemicals (specifically LPS) to enter into her bloodstream, contributing to her fatigue and pain. Four weeks into her gluten elimination diet she started noticing an improvement.

TOP TIP

Consider a six-week trial of eliminating gluten and/or dairy to see whether an improvement in fatigue or pain occurs before reintroducing it gradually. This would mean stopping breads/crackers/wraps/most baked goods and replacing them with gluten-free options from your local supermarket, fresh fruit/legumes, and grains such as quinoa/buckwheat and steel cut oats.

Other pro-inflammatory foods

Polyamines: An excess of polyamine intake can increase the nervous system sensitivity, which can amplify pain. Reducing polyamines can help in improving pre-existing pain sensitivity. Orange juice often contains high levels of polyamines so it may be worthwhile considering reducing the amount you consume, especially carbonated or fizzy ones due to the combination of high sugar and high polyamines. Potato, especially as processed crisps, also contains high levels of polyamines.

Caffeine: On the one hand, caffeine can improve pain when combined with other analgesics. However, caffeine disturbs sleep and if you therefore have a combination of chronic pain and sleep disturbances then pain is likely to be worsened if you have coffee. One suggestion is to not have any caffeine at least seven to eight hours before the intended time of sleep.

High-fructose corn syrup: Overall sugar in any form is very inflammatory and any modifications of sugar, such as fructose or high-fructose corn syrup, are all inflammatory. It is present ubiquitously in most foodstuffs and quite often exceedingly difficult to avoid.

Excitotoxins: These are small amino acid molecules often added to food to enhance flavour and improve taste. These food additives stimulate some nerve cells and cause excitation. The concern is that in some patients it can become excessive or prolonged. Consumption of such foodstuffs that are rich in these toxins can cause nervous system changes.

The two main excitotoxins commonly used are glutamate and aspartate, which act as excitatory neurotransmitters, and there are case reports linking these to worsening pain and other neurological issues like headaches, migraine-like episodes, seizures and behaviour changes. In 2001, a study described the history of four women who had been diagnosed to have fibromyalgia. All these women had the condition for almost 17 years and they had been thoroughly investigated for everything else. All of them responded very well to diets that had no monosodium glutamate (MSG) or aspartate in their diet.

Aspartame is a common constituent of low-calorie sweeteners, sugar-free sweets and gum. Glutamate is often seen in products that contain MSG, yeast extract, gelatin, textured protein and hydrolysed protein, carrageenan, soy protein isolate and whey protein concentrate. In fact, a good rule of thumb is that the more a food is processed, the higher the concentration and likelihood that it contains MSG.

Other pro-inflammatory foods to consider avoiding/reducing, especially if you are in pain due to central sensitisation, are:

- Red meat, including processed versions such as hamburgers.
- Certain oils and fats that come from soybean/safflower/corn and sunflower.
- White bread, rice and corn cereals.
- Fizzy drinks, including diet, and fruit juice, energy drinks and flavourings.
- Sweets and biscuits/cakes/pastries/doughnuts/pies and sugary desserts.

Which foods do you eat regularly – pro- or anti-inflammatory foods? Can you decide on two pro-inflammatory foods you can give up over the next two weeks to see if they make a difference to your pain?

PESTICIDES

A huge number of pesticides are now being used to grow big yields of fresh produce. This is now becoming a systemic problem. It means that washing your vegetables and fruits isn't going to be enough as every part of the produce probably absorbs the pesticide and therefore passes into us. This has implications as we cannot be sure whether environmental toxins are contributing to some pain conditions and sensitising the nervous and immune systems.

The Environmental Working Group (EWG) is a US non-profit organisation and it produces an annual list of 12 dirty products and 15 clean products by estimating the amount of pesticide in them.[23] Take a look at the list below, last updated in 2020, and see if you can go for the cleaner produce. This has been broadly adopted by the UK as well.[24]

Dirty Dozen™	Clean Fifteen™
Strawberries, nectarines, apples, grapes, peaches, cherries, pears, tomatoes, spinach, kale, celery, potatoes	Avocados, sweet corn, pineapple, onions, papaya, frozen sweet peas, aubergines, asparagus, cauliflower, cantaloupe melon, broccoli, mushrooms, cabbage, honeydew melon, kiwi

Adding in anti-inflammatory foods

While there are several foodstuffs that are now proven to be anti-inflammatory, a broad approach would be a healthy diet that incorporates all this.

The **Mediterranean diet**, which is high in vegetables, fruits, whole grains, legumes, nuts and seeds with olive oil, is a very safe and effective healthy diet. Red meat consumption and dairy products are limited, with fish and poultry consumed more often.

An **alkaline diet** is rich in fruits, vegetables, seeds, nuts, fish, natural yoghurt, beans and legumes, and is the preferred choice if you are in pain. This is because processed foods and high glycaemic index foods make our bodies more acidic.

Anti-inflammatory carbohydrates

There are some low-density cellular carbohydrates, such as sweet potatoes, carrots or parsnips, which are quite useful to consume as part of a low-carbohydrate diet.

Anti-inflammatory fats

Omega-3 unsaturated fatty acids are anti-inflammatory so reduce the amount of omega-6 you consume and increase your dietary intake of omega-3. Omega-3 is noted to have the ability to inhibit microglia activation, thus further reducing inflammation in the brain. High levels of omega-3 are found in fish, especially cold-water fish such as mackerel, herring and salmon, as well as in other foods like flaxseed and almonds. Switching to olive oil is a good way to increase your omega-3 intake.

ANTI-INFLAMMATORY FOODS

- Whole grains: wholegrain bread, oats (steel cut), brown rice, barley, bulgur wheat, quinoa, couscous, polenta and rye bread.
- Beans/nuts/seeds: black beans, kidney beans, chickpeas, hummus, nuts and seeds like walnuts, almonds, pecans and peanuts, sunflower seeds, flaxseed, pumpkin seeds and legumes like edamame beans and sugar snap peas.
- Fruits: berries, cherries and dark-coloured fruits.

- Vegetables: peppers, tomatoes, spinach, kale, leaf lettuce, mixed greens, dark and leafy greens, broccoli, sprouts, cauliflower, radishes and cucumbers.
- Oils: olive and coconut oil.
- Fish: preferably cold-water fish including salmon, herring, anchovies, sardines and mackerel.
- Tea: black tea, green tea, white tea and herbal tea.
- Chocolate: dark chocolate >70% cocoa.
- Wine: red wine (no more than 14 units a week).
- Sources of fibre: raspberries, blueberries, avocado, broccoli, nuts, seeds, beans, cauliflower, kale and apples.

Could nutrition changes help you with chronic pain? Make notes here for you to discuss with your doctor:

_____

_____

_____

Ensure adequate hydration

While not causally related to pain, a number of my fibromyalgia and chronic fatigue patients have found it quite useful to ensure that hydration is maintained. It reduces their fatigue, clears up their fibro fog and they feel that it improves energy and concentration. It was one of the recommendations that Sarah was given and it helped her. She was told to have a couple of glasses in the morning and then a glass with each meal and another couple before going to bed.

While the evidence is lacking on an upper limit, popular suggestions and discussions with nutritionists and other doctors suggest that we should be having between 1 and 1.5 litres per day.

How much water do you drink? Is this something you could improve over the next few weeks?

Essential nutrients and multivitamins

Another problem of highly processed foods and the takeaway culture is the reduction in essential nutrients and various vitamins. Vitamin deficiencies can contribute to chronic pain and mood disorders. A balanced quantity of vitamins and minerals are needed and, if natural food does not have enough, then the use of multivitamins and other supplements needs to be considered (see below).[25]

- **Vitamin A** is best taken as beta-carotene and helps in detoxifying certain harmful substances. Carotenoids can be another source of vitamin A.
- **Vitamin B** is a complex of eight vitamins with B12 being most relevant for pain worsening, especially when it is deficient. Vitamin B2 can be useful in migraine relief and vitamin B6 in premenstrual cramps.
- **Vitamin C** is a powerful antioxidant and is needed for muscle and ligament repair. Since humans cannot make vitamin C on their own, it does need to come from external sources.

- **Vitamin D** (sunshine vitamin) is required for about 200 genes in the body to function well. It also helps in boosting the immune system, preventing diabetes and muscle strength. Most populations are deficient in vitamin D and deficiency can often cause widespread pain. In my practice, when I see patients who have a diagnosis of fibromyalgia, I always recommend supplementation of vitamin D if it is even borderline low.
- **Vitamins E and K** act as antioxidants so have powerful anti-inflammatory effects.
- Minerals like **calcium** are often useful for bone strength alongside vitamin D, and low calcium can often cause muscle pain.
- **Magnesium** is hugely important for the energy factories of our cells (mitochondria). Low magnesium can worsen muscle pain and cause weakness. It can help in IBS, improve sleep and reduce pain.
- **Chromium, iodine** and **iron** are other trace minerals that are becoming increasingly important to consider supplementing. While the evidence is still being developed, deficiencies of these trace elements can worsen pain or diabetes control.
- **Zinc** and **selenium** both have antioxidant properties and are increasingly recommended for pain conditions.

Supplements[26]

Various supplements that have become increasingly popular in pain management include glucosamine and chondroitin (though evidence has been patchy). Apart from the vitamins above, omega-3 fish oils can help in a variety of pain conditions. Turmeric, ginger, S-adenosylmethionin (SAM) and processed butterbur (a shrub – see page 58) all have anti-inflammatory properties and are increasingly used for conditions like migraine and osteoarthritis.

Antioxidants

Apart from the vitamins mentioned above, other antioxidants also have anti-inflammatory effects. A broad umbrella term for them is 'polyphenols' and they are found in a variety of foods, especially in the skins of fruits and vegetables.

- **L-glutamine** improves neuropathic pain by promoting the body's antioxidant production.
- **Quercetin** is plant-based and acts as an antioxidant and anti-inflammatory.
- **CoQ10** is required by our mitochondria and acts as a powerful antioxidant.
- **N-acetyl cysteine** and **alpha lipoic acid** are other antioxidants that work in the liver to protect and detoxify a variety of substances and protect the muscle, nerve cells and liver.
- **Resveratrol** is usually formed when plants are under attack by insects or an infection. It's found in the skin of red grapes and mulberries and also in red wine.
- **Anthocyanins** are found in blueberry skins and cherries and can also help in reducing pain.

Overall, the aim is to eat more vitamins by consuming lots of fresh vegetables, more coloured and leafy vegetables and less red meat. In short, eat a rainbow diet.

ANTIOXIDANT-RICH FOODS[27]

Spices	Cloves, oregano, ginger, cinnamon, turmeric, basil
Berries/ fruits	Blackberries, cranberries, raspberries, strawberries, blueberries, sour cherries, pomegranate, red grapes, plums, kiwi, prunes
Nuts/ seeds	Walnuts, pecans, flaxseed, sunflower seeds, pistachios
Vegetables	Kale, red cabbage, spinach, artichokes, broccoli
Other	Dark chocolate, red wine, green tea, coffee

Probiotics, prebiotics and synbiotics

- **Probiotics** are essentially living bacteria that can supposedly increase health benefits when consumed by mouth. They have tremendous potential for modifying the gut microbiota, but this is hampered by the fact that we do not know how much or what to take or how much of these bacteria get to various parts of the intestine. Nevertheless, there are a lot of studies that will give us more information in the next few years.
- **Prebiotics**, on the other hand, are considered as additional support or an alternative to probiotics. They could benefit patients with chronic pain, but it is not yet being fully shown to work in humans. Some trials

have been done in patients with stomach disorders, but we still don't have any particular approved drug.

- **Synbiotics** are a combination of the live bacteria and synthetic products (prebiotic and probiotic) and hence they are called synbiotics. They improve the survival of the live bacteria and improve overall health.

ON THE HORIZON: FAECAL MICROBIOTA TRANSPLANTATION

Faecal microbiota transplantation is exactly as it sounds. It's an infusion of faeces that is filtered from a healthy donor and then given as a suppository into the gut of a pain patient to treat certain pain conditions.

It is primarily been done for clostridium difficile diarrhoea and has also been trialled for inflammatory bowel disease, obesity and insulin resistance. There is also a study reporting a pain patient with fibromyalgia who had a full recovery following such a transplant.[28]

While this is still in the early stages, there seem to be many mechanisms that have shown why this strategy could be of importance and of benefit, and therefore there is a possibility that this will become a promising approach to treat chronic pain, especially when it is due to intestinal disorders.

Time of eating

This has been a focus of active research in the last few years and can be anti-inflammatory for a couple of reasons. In a very counter-intuitive study and what the author, Satchin Panda, neuroscientist at the Salk Institute, describes as an 'earth-shattering' moment, it is possible that when we eat is more important than what we eat.[29]

The intestinal clock is regulated by our body's master clock (see page 195) and therefore it gets ready with its digestive juices and the good bacteria in the daytime. It also regulates the release of other enzymes to break down harmful products and eliminate them after it gets the signal that the last meal has been completed.

However, researchers have found that in our modern day and age, if we keep eating for up to 16 to 17 hours, then the intestinal clock never gets the chance to repair and heal the damaged cells in our intestine wall. It needs at least 12 to 16 hours of empty time to do this.

In a fascinating experiment, Panda and his team proved this by taking two identical groups of mice. One group were fed the standard Western diet, full of processed food and calories, randomly through the day, while the other group were given the same food but within a window of 8 to 12 hours.

When they saw how the mice fared at the end of 18 weeks, they were shocked to find that those that ate randomly for long durations of time were morbidly 'obese' (in mice grams) and sick from a variety of diseases, while those from the second group remained healthy. They then took the obese unwell mice and allowed them to eat, but now within the window of 8 to 12 hours, and they regained their health.

They repeated this study by looking at the eating habits of a group of human volunteers. Not surprisingly, many people were eating for more than 15 hours of the day. They asked a cohort of this group of people to eat their portions within a

10-hour window, meaning a 14-hour fast if possible.[30] The volunteers reported weight loss and better circadian rhythms, better mood and more energy within three to four months.

This is one of the reasons why intermittent fasting techniques and time-restricted feeding, which call for fasting periods of 12 to 16 hours, and sometimes longer, are becoming popular.

Intermittent fasting diet

A fasting mimicking diet is a variety of low-calorie, high-fat diet that dampens microglial activation and protects the nerves. This protection and reduction in inflammation can reduce pain. By giving a 12-hour window of rest to our gut, the nervous and immune systems get the chance to clear up, repair and clean out the intestine, almost a self-repair process. What we are doing is giving a period of rest to the intestine to facilitate that. If we fast for longer durations i.e. more than 14–16 hours in a day, we would then be producing more ketone bodies, which also dampen inflammation and improve concentration.

The period of fasting not only reduces inflammation in the intestine and brain, it also allows organs like the liver to detoxify and eliminate any harmful products that would have built up during the day. The analogy I tell my patients is the turnaround time that hotels have between room occupants. Usually they need about two to four hours to make the room spotless and clean. In our body's case, it is around 10–12 hours – the longer the time you give (the more hours of fasting) the more the body not only cleans up but also gets to repair and rejuvenate various cells and tissues. This not only has a pain-relieving effect, but can be useful in many other medical conditions and for general health and ageing.

> **TOP TIP**
>
> Choose a 10–12-hour window that fits your lifestyle and trial the technique. You can still have water, green tea or black coffee during the fast period.

Summary

- Aim for a wider variety of plant-based foods to ensure a greater degree of biodiversity for the microbiome. A whole food, plant-based diet is most ideal with low quantities of low-fat meat and adequate fish.
- Consider incorporating high-antioxidant and high-fibre food that can nourish your good bacteria and use cooking oils that are rich in omega-3, such as flaxseed, walnut or olive oil.
- Avoid repeated exposure to antibiotics, which can affect the diversity of the microbiome and contribute to further pain.
- Pay special attention to your diet during times of stress, when we will often reach out for the ultra-processed foods as they act on the reward centre to ease symptoms.
- Take care during critical periods. There are three times in our life when the gut–microbiota–brain axis is at risk of being significantly altered: the period through pregnancy to the first few years of life, during early adulthood (17–25 years) and in old age. This means that there are large periods when we can make changes to our pain through diet.

- Aim to reduce your consumption of animal fat, especially the processed meat that is often the staple of most fast food outlets.
- Avoid mass-produced and processed food as much as possible.
- Eat more fermented foods and probiotics. Fermented foods like kimchi, kombucha, sauerkraut, kefir and naturally fermented and unpasteurised foodstuffs are excellent sources of probiotics.
- Consider supplements. Ginger, vitamin D and curcumin in foods have been shown to have some benefit in muscle pain. In arthritis, use of probiotics along with omega-3 fatty acids and turmeric extract has been shown to be useful.
- Eat together with family/friends. It has been shown that eating with someone else can make the mealtime pleasant and improve the social feeling of well-being.

CHAPTER 7

Sleep

*A full night of sleep . . . . that most powerful elixir of
wellness and vitality, dispensed through every conceivable
biological pathway.*

Matthew Walker, *How to Sleep*

SEAN HAS BEEN leading the way as a patient advocate for people
in pain and has been on various peer support and patient safety
groups in Cornwall. His national profile has seen him travel to
the House of Lords in 2019 to present his story of what life
was like on pain medication. Just three years ago, however,
Sean had passed 25 years of being on high-dose opioids and all
manner of nerve pain drugs, and was almost a social recluse.
He had a hernia repair at the age of 32 and had been left with
nerve damage in the scar around the mesh.

I spoke to Sean recently and he recollected how he went for
what he thought would be a straightforward day case hernia
repair. Unfortunately for him, he had an immediate onset of
nerve pain after the first surgery. They thought that it was
because of the scar and he underwent a further two surgical
explorations to see if the nerve could be released from the scar.
Ultimately, it was decided that no further surgery was possible
and that he had to live his life with the pain.

'It was an opioid oblivion for me,' Sean said. 'I was popping pills all the time. I was on duloxetine, nortriptyline, gabapentin and finally 160mg per day of morphine along with liquid morphine. Nothing seemed to work. The worst was the complete inability to sleep and have any quality of life. I couldn't sleep for more than a couple of hours before the pain would wake me up.'

Sean described how he kept going from surgeon to surgeon and was then referred to the pain clinic. He had trials of numerous pain medications and strong opioids. Going from being really fit and healthy and someone who prided himself on being an active waterskier, keen tennis player and sailor, to someone who was unable to go out of the house on most days and help out in any capacity at home for any length of time, was a big frustration for him. His function and quality of life all suffered.

We know that sleep can often get interrupted because of pain. However, it is now more than two years since Sean has come off all his medications. With a combination of mindfulness and exercise/breathing techniques, he is able to sleep for more than seven hours every night. He is aware of the pain but, as he says, he put it 'in the back of his wardrobe'. He is not on any sleeping tablets nor is he on pain medications.

How is this possible? What exactly is the relationship between sleep and pain?

While it may seem intuitive to you that pain would obviously interrupt and cause sleeplessness, the research shows that often it isn't pain that causes loss of sleep. Sometimes it can be the other way around. In this chapter I will show you why optimising sleep is a particularly important strategy for achieving the pain-free mindset and reducing your pain.

Firstly, let's do a mini sleep assessment to see if you have a possible sleep problem:[1]

	Yes	No
Do you sleep fewer than 7 hours or more than 9 hours on weekdays?		
Do you sleep fewer than 7 hours or more than 9 hours on weekends?		
Is there more than an hour's difference between your weekday and weekend sleep duration?		
Do you wake up unrefreshed?		
Do you have naps longer than 30 minutes during the daytime?		
Do you drink less than 1 litre of water during the day?		
Do you go to bed stressed/angry/upset often?		
Do you watch TV or eat in bed?		
Do you drink caffeine/alcohol within 3 hours of bedtime?		

There is an important link between sleep and pain. Having less than one hour's difference between your weekday and weekend sleep is considered good, with seven to nine hours recommended for any sleep time. How do you fare?

If you answered 'Yes' to three or more of the questions above then there is a good chance that optimising your sleep can improve your overall ability to overcome pain.

The Importance of Sleep

There have been some remarkable advances that have changed how we view sleep and its place in our evolution. We have generally thought that sleep helps to refresh us, but we never really knew what was happening in this process. We sleep for almost a third of our lives and we now understand that sleep has many other important life-nourishing roles to play.

Like in the field of medicine, there has been some excellent research and understanding of the brain and the role of sleep over the last 10–15 years, which means our knowledge of

SLEEP AS A FOUNDATION

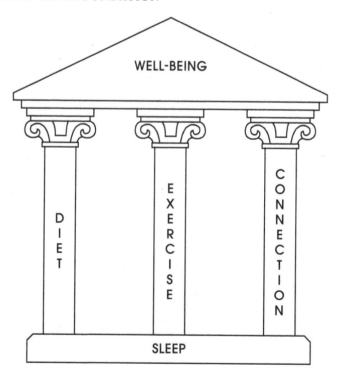

what exactly happens to the body and the mind during sleep is exponentially much better. In fact, according to Matthew Walker, author of *Why We Sleep*, sleep can often become a fundamental foundation stone on top of which the pillars of diet, exercise and social connections can be placed.[2]

Multiple studies over the years have now confirmed that sleep and its duration is vital, and that reduced duration of sleep on an extended basis – the bane of our modern light-filled life – can actually be life-shortening.

While most organisations, including the WHO, have advised at least eight hours of sleep every night, almost two-thirds of adults in developed countries don't achieve that. Fewer than six hours of sleep on a daily basis affects the immune and nervous systems negatively, thus putting us at risk of heart disease and Alzheimer's.

Walker asserts that a good eight hours of sleep:

- Enhances our ability to learn and memorise.
- Recharges our emotional circuits and networks.
- Allows us to dream where we can make sense of our past experiences and present knowledge, improving creativity.
- Recharges our immune system.
- Restores our metabolic and hormone levels like insulin.
- Lowers our blood pressure and reduces stress.
- Fine-tunes our microbiome health.

Sleep and the glymphatic system

One of the more important reasons for the proposed seven to nine hours of sleep is the understanding and presence of a lymphatic system that exists within the brain. It's common knowledge that the body has a lymphatic system to remove waste products that build up in various tissues in the body. Junctions of these lymphatic systems are known as lymph nodes and are found in various parts of the body.

However, it was always a bit of a mystery how the brain removes its waste products. We now know that the brain has its own lymphatic system formed by the glial cells (yep, the same housekeeper cells from previous chapters) called the glymphatic system. This helps to remove the waste products of metabolism over the course of the day.

Glial cells are present between and around the neurons in the brain. They can decrease in size by as much as 60 per cent when we sleep so that there can be an efficient waste clearance of the products from that area. Imagine a situation where there has been a very raucous football match and the cleaners have to clean the stadium after the game; hard work you might think. Imagine if there was a power to shrink the seats by 60 per cent! How much easier it would be to achieve a complete clean of the stadium, and not to mention time-saving. That is how the glymphatic system does its job. And it needs time – not three to four hours, but seven to nine.

Sleep Cycles

If you slept for a typical eight-hour period of undisturbed sleep then your sleep would go through various stages called sleep cycles.

Broadly there are two phases of sleep: a phase where rapid eye movement is observed, called REM sleep, and another known as non-REM (NREM) sleep. The NREM phase is

TYPICAL SLEEP ARCHITECTURE

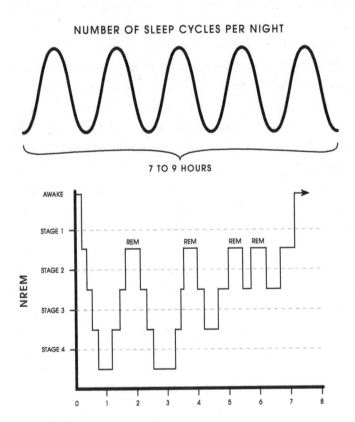

NUMBER OF SLEEP CYCLES PER NIGHT

7 TO 9 HOURS

further divided into four stages, with the fourth stage being the deepest sleep.

There are generally around five cycles through an eight-hour period each night. Each cycle lasts about 90 minutes. The usual division between REM and NREM is 20:80 in a particular cycle, but in the first half, more time is spent in NREM sleep, so if you sleep later at night, then NREM sleep gets sacrificed. The importance of this loss will become clearer later in this chapter.

REM only occupies one-fifth of the time spent in a 8 hour period (<2 hours) and it is often the phase of sleep where dreams occur. Researchers feel that dreaming is not just something that happens, but is an important facet of the activity that the brain does as part of its duty to maintain equilibrium and good function.

How pain interferes with REM and NREM

NREM is needed to eliminate or take out unnecessary connections between nerves that have formed during the day, whereas REM sleep is able to reinforce other connections and can strengthen them.

In the context of chronic pain, this understanding of sleep cycles is very important. In chronic pain, sleep time and quality is reduced and often the NREM part of the cycle is lost first. Given the role of NREM sleep in removing unwanted nerve connections and synapses, the fact that poor sleep reduces NREM means that unwanted connections and inflammation are allowed to persist. Sleep often never goes down to stages three or four, so the deeper phases of NREM sleep – which are essential for the brain and body to repair and refresh at the cellular level – progressively get reduced. Research has found that in conditions like fibromyalgia and widespread pain, there is a specific lack of slow wave sleep, or the deep stages three and four, and other phases.[3]

This lack of restorative sleep in chronic pain patients can explain the memory issues like forgetfulness that often occur, and could also explain the fatigue, brain fog and the pain that these patients experience.

One study looked at sleep quality in 121 chronic pain patients from Austria. The researchers found that more than 60 per cent reported fragmented sleep with almost 30 per cent having slept fewer than five hours, and close to 40 per cent having a delayed onset of sleep, which meant that they needed to move around in bed for almost 30 minutes before falling asleep.[4]

What they found was that sleep quality is significantly affected in patients suffering with chronic pain. Psychological factors and the way the patients experienced their pain also significantly influenced the association between pain and sleep quality. This shows that psychological factors and their management can have a significant impact on the association between pain and sleep.

The reciprocal nature of the relationship between pain and sleep has been studied by researchers who looked at 18 studies and concluded that sleep problems usually occur earlier and can increase the risk of chronic pain.[5] What is hopeful to note is that it is possible to improve any of this by simply improving the quality and duration of sleep.

SLEEP DEPRIVATION AND PAIN

With regards to sleep deprivation, it is now getting clearer from the evidence that, when we deprive someone of sleep, we increase their pain sensitivity. When researchers conducted a forced awakening study in 2015, they compared patients who were randomly woken up through the night to those who had fewer hours of sleep but at least slept continuously. Overall, both groups slept for a total of 280 minutes while being awake for 200 minutes. Patients who were woken up randomly experienced worse pain than the other group, indicating that loss of the sleep cycles has a worse effect.[6]

The relationship between pain and sleep

Sleep complaints are present in more than 60 per cent of pain patients, and those with arthritic conditions have sleep problems more often, while 50 per cent of patients with insomnia have chronic pain.[7] The nature of the sleep disturbance can include fragmentation of sleep, a decrease in the efficiency of sleep and reduced slow wave sleep.[8]

Poor sleep can be due to a variety of reasons, such as:

- difficulty initiating sleep
- disrupted sleep
- early morning waking
- unrefreshed sleep

Pain can amplify or actually cause all of the problems above. The relationship between sleep and pain is bidirectional in the sense that poor sleep can bring on pain and sometimes sleep disorders can be there for years before pain comes along.

Disturbed sleep patterns are very common. It is sometimes thought, certainly in medicolegal settings, that disturbances in sleep patterns occur many months to years before a diagnosis of chronic pain conditions like fibromyalgia.[9] Certainly, unrefreshed sleep is one of the cardinal signs of that condition and will contribute to the worsening of pain. A study of almost 15,000 Norwegian women showed that sleep disorders can predict the development of widespread pain and fibromyalgia 10 years later.[10] Overall the research seems to suggest that sleep disturbances may predict pain to a greater degree than pain predicting sleep. If anything, poor sleep can make the experience of pain much worse.

A key trend in studies of large populations is that disturbed sleep can predict new occurrences and flare-ups of chronic pain rather than the other way round. We now very much think that sleep issues can predict pain, which means that if we can rectify our sleep and get better at improving sleep then it should improve, and maybe even prevent, pain as well.

The effect on pain-related sleep loss on the immune system

The nervous system is tightly connected to the immune system and the pain system. This means that disturbed sleep spills over into multiple systems and causes an overactivity of the sympathetic nervous system – the fight and flight system and the stress cortisol system.[11]

While it is an important mechanism that's present in all of us to ensure survival, especially in the acute phase where it causes the release of adrenaline and cortisol to help us, it is not good when it remains active in the long term.

As we saw in Chapter 5, increased stress causes inflammation in the brain, affecting both the body and the brain and thus lowering overall immunity. This has implications: it means that, for example, a flu shot or even the COVID-19 vaccine is likely to generate a greater number of antibodies in our system when we have had a good night's sleep. When sleep is deprived, the immune system is not able to mount a sufficient response and therefore we continue to be at risk of contracting any flu or viral infection.

Hypertension and the risk of heart attacks are increased when there is sleep deprivation. An overactive sympathetic nervous system causes prolonged adrenaline and cortisol to remain in the system. If we can get seven to nine hours of sleep, these changes are reversible and the cycle of the sympathetic system can be cut, increasing growth hormone and reducing cortisol. Apart from pain, decreased sleep increases the risk of type 2 diabetes by making the body less sensitive to insulin, increasing the risk of metabolic syndrome (see page 160).

The good news is that improving your sleep can reverse all of these above changes. A good night's sleep can bring about greater impulse control, reduce your cortisol, calm your sympathetic nervous system, increase the amount of growth hormone and make the cells more sensitive to insulin.

The reason all of this is relevant to pain is that diseases like diabetes, obesity and heart attacks are all potential extra sources of anxiety and are possible causes of chronic pain themselves.

The Master Clock

One of the more important discoveries in sleep medicine has been the finding that not only does every organ have its own clock, but there is a master clock in the brain, which regulates all those clocks. Since we know that sleep disturbances can put you at risk for chronic pain, it's important that you know the factors that can be altered to improve your sleep duration and reduce the risks of chronic pain.

The master clock is an area of the brain called the suprachiasmatic nucleus, which contains just 20,000 neurons and is located in the anterior hypothalamus. There is another structure (which we saw in Chapter 5) called the thalamus, which acts as a big gate for sleep and ensures that it effectively filters out all of the sensations that are continuing to bombard us even as we sleep, from both the external and internal environment. The suprachiasmatic nucleus is also an important centre for the regulation of pain signals and it regulates the pineal gland, which produces the sleep hormone melatonin.[12]

When light hits the retina of the eye, let's say in the morning, it acts on special cells in the retina and they release a chemical called melanopsin. This signals the anterior hypothalamus – and from there the master clock – to start the day. Melatonin gradually rises after the onset of darkness as the eyes get the signal and let the clock know. The clock then triggers the pineal gland to make more melatonin.

Our ability to go to sleep and then sleep well and wake up is governed by two factors: circadian rhythm and sleep pressure. The sleep pressure is caused by a gradual build-up of a chemical called adenosine. Adenosine accumulates in our brains as the day goes on and, once it reaches a critical level, it brings about that phase that we recognise as sleepiness. Often it can lead to an overpowering urge to sleep by a particular time when the levels become high.

When we go to sleep, adenosine gets effectively washed away by the glymphatic system. If sufficient time is not given for sleep, then we wake up still with the adenosine floating about, feeling groggy and tired.

There are people who truly may be able to function on very little sleep and it is now known that this group of people may have genetic variant of BHLHE41 or DEC2 gene.[13] However, most of us do need between seven and nine hours of sleep on most days.

The impact of caffeine

Caffeine essentially acts on the same receptors where adenosine acts. It blocks these receptors and prevents adenosine from locking to them. The caffeine prevents the natural adenosine from bringing about sleeping and you are tricked into staying awake. The caffeine level hits a peak 30 minutes after you have it, but it hangs about for five to seven hours. Eventually, when the caffeine wears off, the amount of adenosine has built up so much that sleep comes on even more powerfully. This is not really helpful in the long term because it is not a natural way of achieving sleep.

Technology and the master clock

If we are exposed to significant amounts of blue light – essentially light from smartphones, laptops or television – then that light activates the retina in the eyes and this tells the master clock that it is still daylight. This affects the circadian rhythm and over time can cause a significant impact on various body systems.

Blue light also interferes with the melatonin release that builds the momentum to sleep. Most smartphones have a setting for blue light blocking and blue light filter glasses are also available for purchase.

AGEING, PAIN AND SLEEP

Old age is a common period when sleep disturbances occur. By 40 years of age, the NREM deep sleep phase

---

starts to go down. In older adults there is almost a 70 per cent reduction in the NREM deep sleep phase.

It's not that older adults do not need sleep, but that they are not able to generate the sleep that's needed. As age increases, the first parts of the brain that are often affected are the frontal regions, where sleep is generated. Having chronic pain accelerates all these changes, thus affecting sleep much more.

Screening for Sleep Problems

There are a number of tools that pain clinics and other specialist respiratory and sleep services use for screening. The Pittsburgh Sleep Quality Index (PSQI) is an approved research and self-scoring tool to see how much your pain has been interfering with your life. Other tools are the Satisfaction, Alertness, Timing, Efficiency and Duration (SATED) questionnaire and the Epworth Sleepiness Scale. The NHS also provides a tool for self-assessment (see page 311).

Polysomnography is a comprehensive recording of all the changes that occur during sleep and is usually performed at night in a special laboratory. It monitors many body functions including eye movements, muscle activities, snoring and ECG and EEG during sleep. It allows us to get a good idea of the overall body functions during the time of sleep and it can help identify certain sleep disorders. However, polysomnograms (sleep studies) are very rarely done for people in pain with disturbed sleep in the UK.

A sleep study can be considered if:

- you are having frequent disruptions in your sleep, or
- you have episodes of daytime drowsiness, or
- you experience unusual movements during sleep, or
- your partner reports that you snore excessively, or
- you have difficulty falling or staying asleep.

These sleep studies are often done by respiratory departments and you would need to speak to your GP or specialist regarding this.

Monitoring Sleep

The Sleep Council in the UK provides an impartial service and raises the awareness of the importance of a good night's sleep for health and well-being. It provides a good 30-day sleep plan and sleep hygiene tips that are very useful to try (see page 312).

Self-monitoring

There are numerous phone apps (see pages 311–312) that help track your sleep, though sleep trackers are not for everyone. They are, at this point in time, not as technologically accurate as a sleep study would be, so they are not useful for a diagnosis of any sleep problems. They can't read your actual brainwaves so they use surrogate measures like movement, ultrasound waves, sound detection or heart rate, and then compare those to an algorithm and arrive at a conclusion. If you are a perfectionist and therefore watch the numbers too carefully, sleep trackers may not be for you.

An actigraph is a validated electronic instrument that is often available in the form of a wrist watch and can be used to monitor sleep and circadian rhythms. It does help in gathering useful information that can be used as part of treatment.

Psychophysiological arousal

This is a very fancy way of considering the fact that when someone is anxious there is an increased amount of sympathetic nervous system activity, and this will mean that there is often an increased amount of adrenaline, which will reduce the blood flow to the skin in general. This means that if skin temperature is measured it would reflect cooler skin readings. The core temperature has to be low for you to fall asleep. Conversely, if the peripheral temperatures are low, which means the body hasn't lost its heat and the core remains high, then it ends up taking longer for the patient to fall asleep and they also report higher pain levels.

Treatments for Sleep

If pain management is to infuse hope, then improving sleep is a vital part of the plan. Unfortunately, all of the good benefits of sleep get taken away when you have persistent pain and so it is vital to address this from the outset of your diagnosis and adopt supportive strategies that will combine lifestyle changes with non-drug therapies, and certain drugs when deemed suitable.

The core of the problem is often a hypersensitive nervous system with neuroinflammation and this can happen for a variety of reasons (see Chapter 6). Therefore, if we are to solve the sleep issue, we need to calm the nervous system to a point where it can respond to the body's commands.

Medications

There are several drugs that can be used or trialled for promoting sleep.[14] Unfortunately, in the UK, none of these drugs are recommended long term because they interrupt or disrupt sleep patterns much more. However, if you are having a particularly stressful time, they may be options to discuss with your GP/pain specialist. Common drugs used are:

Amitriptyline

This has a side effect of causing night-time sedation and therefore can improve sleep in the short term. One of the things to remember with most medications, including antidepressants like amitriptyline, is that they can sometimes exacerbate other mood disturbances and worsen quality of life. Unfortunately, antidepressant drugs, in the long run, can actually disrupt the sleep wave patterns on EEG and increase the number of night awakenings.

Zopiclone/zolpidem

These are useful in acute situations of insomnia, but they can be habit-forming and hence GPs may prescribe them only for short durations of time. It has been shown that the kind of brainwaves that occur during these drug-induced sleeps are very different and not what the human body needs to have the usual restorative effects of sleep. They also have a number of side effects, such as grogginess or fogginess, memory problems and sometimes the risk of amnesia. The worst and most dangerous side effects are the impact of the drug on attention skills and driving, and this is due to the slowing of reaction times.

These drugs increase the risk of having a feature called 'rebound insomnia', which is when patients risk suffering far worse sleep deprivation when they stop the drug after a five-day course, and this can become a vicious cycle.

Many studies have now been done comparing the effectiveness of these medications to placebo and they have shown that they are very slightly more effective than the placebo pill.[15] Both the drugs and the placebo seemed to reduce the time it took patients to fall asleep and effectively the drugs only produce a very slight improvement in subjective sleep patterns, but the risk of harm was much higher compared to non-drug therapies.

TOP TIPS WITH MEDICATIONS

- It is important to discuss any of these medication options with your consultant as well as your GP before trialling any of them. The reality is that no medication right now exists on the market that is safe and effective enough to induce natural sleep.
- Older medications like diazepam and amitriptyline sedate rather than induce natural sleep. In that sense they are not very different from alcohol.
- Zolpidem and zopiclone can cause an element of dependence and they work for only short periods of time, so are maximally prescribed for three to five days. The longer you take them, the more they tend to disrupt the natural sleep patterns that are very important.
- Trying to improve sleep using medications is at best a short-term strategy and at worst no better than taking a placebo.[16]

- Drug-induced sleep causes a weakening of the nerve circuits and interferes with the ability to learn to the extent that it could very well be a risk for memory loss.
- There is now compelling evidence that using prescription sleep drugs is linked to a higher chance of developing cancer and earlier mortality. **Patients taking sleeping pills were roughly 4.6 times more likely to die over a 2.5-year period compared to those who did not.**[17] This could be due to increased infections due to the effect on the immune system or side effect-related accidents.

Melatonin

Melatonin is produced by the pineal gland and its release is tightly regulated. It is dependent on the master clock going off in the brain for it to go into action. Melatonin increases as the evening gets darker and peaks in the middle of sleep, before gradually reducing by daybreak. Melatonin induces the sedation – it is often the starter gun for the race – and it lowers the core body temperature thus creating the conditions for initiating sleep. If you are wondering why melatonin is not prescribed regularly it is exactly because of this – it is an indicator to tell the body to prepare for sleep, but it has no role in keeping you asleep.

Although it has very few side effects and is inexpensive, the evidence is not significant enough for use on the NHS. If you do wish to trial it, dosages range from 1 to 5mg taken about 45 minutes before bedtime. Melatonin gradually decreases as ageing occurs so it is much more useful in the elderly age group.

Mind-body therapies

Since sleep disturbance often occurs in symptom clusters with pain and possibly fatigue, it makes sense to think of broad strategies that can work on multiple clusters rather than just one symptom. Mind–body interventions have become quite popular in this regard because they provide patients with other knowledge and skills, are often relatively inexpensive and can be combined with other medication strategies with minimal side effects.

A large body of studies was reviewed looking specifically at which mind–body interventions helped with symptom clusters of sleep deprivation.[18] Meditation, music and virtual reality were compared with respect to efficacy for pain fatigue and sleep disturbance. The researchers found that CBT and hypnosis training produced improvements in all symptoms individually, while relaxation improved pain and sleep disturbance. Music therapy improved pain and fatigue while meditation-based interventions improved fatigue and sleep disturbance. Much like in pain management, behavioural methods such as CBT have shown to be as effective as and in some cases more effective than drugs.

Cognitive behavioural therapy for insomnia (CBTI)

The evidence now favouring this behavioural technique is so significant that mainstream organisations like the American College of Physicians have made this the first line treatment for all individuals with insomnia and not drugs, which is a landmark change.[19]

It can be delivered as a group or individually in person or online. Components of the programme would include such techniques as relaxation techniques or training, which is complemented by biofeedback, coping skills training, increasing activity levels and goal setting. Newer therapies also include the addition of some movement-based strategies along with acceptance and commitment therapy (ACT) and mindfulness. With the help of a therapist, patients are given certain behavioural techniques that are individualised for them. The ultimate aim is about breaking or attempting to change bad sleep habits and address any sleep-inhibiting factors, anxieties or emotional changes.

Mindfulness-based meditation

This is one of the most useful mind–body therapies that has shown in research to improve sleep-related problems. A new study by Spanish sleep scientists has shown that mindfulness-based meditation can improve the quality of sleep in fibromyalgia patients and that these benefits lasted even at the three-month follow-up visit.[20]

Bathing and other rituals

Several studies have looked into balneotherapy for the treatment of painful conditions like fibromyalgia.[21] Balneotherapy, which means bathing to treat an illness, appears to reduce stiffness and pain. This isn't surprising given that warm water helps to reduce muscle tension, promotes relaxation and lessens overall pain.

Electrical neuromodulation

There are electrical magnetic and auditory stimulation methods for boosting deep sleep quality. However, they are still in the early developmental stages.

Sleep Hygiene

As previously mentioned, poor sleep patterns often precede the onset of pain. The American Sleep Foundation has produced a comprehensive document highlighting the dos and don'ts for good sleep hygiene (see Resources, page 312).[22] Many of these are not just beneficial for general health, but they can also reduce the overall impact of poor sleep on pain and can help if pain is preventing you from falling asleep, disturbing your sleep or waking you up. Some of the top tips include:

Routine

It is important to keep a very consistent sleep schedule so that the brain effectively can be retrained to know when it is time to sleep, even during weekends. Aim for seven to nine hours of sleep each day. It is also important to have a cycle and a pattern of winding down and relaxing for at least a couple of hours in the evening before going to bed. Consider a regular pre-bed habit, such as taking a warm shower or bath, reading a book, listening to some bedtime music or doing some light stretching. Initially reduce the amount of time spent in bed if you're not feeling sleepy. This allows the body to start to build up more adenosine and that increases the sleep pressure so that when you do fall asleep, you do so naturally and for longer. If you cannot sleep, get up, go to a different room and return when you feel sleepy.

Avoid long naps

Taking long naps late in the day may interfere with your ability to sleep well at night. However, it is fine to lie down for 10 minutes or so to relax when you are feeling overwhelmed, and a short nap of 20–30 minutes can help to improve mood, alertness and performance.

Exercise

One of the most important things to consider is exercise. I know that this can be quite difficult for pain patients. Many studies prove that exercising on a daily basis can be quite efficient in improving sleep quality (see Chapter 8 for more on this). Aim for at least 30 minutes of activity each day. Finish any physical activity at least three hours before sleep time and avoid strenuous workouts (not including sex!) close to bedtime.

Diet and nutrition

Dietary supplements such as vitamin D can be quite useful in improving overall pain and sleep patterns. Avoid any coffee or caffeine at least six to eight hours before you plan to sleep and ensure adequate hydration during the day (see page 174). Avoid high-sodium, heavy, spicy or fried foods or excessive fluids close to sleep time, and avoid alcohol within three hours of bedtime. Try to eliminate any after-dinner snacking.

Quiet environment

Create a quiet environment and make the bedroom as dark as possible. Keep the temperature cool (18–20°C) and use your bedroom only for sleep and sex. When possible, try to avoid emotionally upsetting conversations and activities before attempting to sleep.

Complementary therapies

Consider using complementary therapy, such as gentle massage, deep breathing or relaxation techniques, all of which will soothe the brain and enable it to proceed to peaceful sleep. All of these create a wind-down effect for the brain.

Circadian rhythm reset

Ensure adequate exposure to natural light as it helps to maintain a healthy sleep–wake cycle. My patients have found that when they get up in the morning, exposing themselves to just ten minutes of natural sunlight or even a light box for the first hour of waking can establish a circadian rhythm. The circadian rhythm can also be stabilised with either a short walk or some light exercise during the day. Decrease the lighting at night by using warm spectrum lights (2500Kelvin) and switching off any unnecessary lights.

Digital detox

I would also recommend that all mobile devices are switched off at least 90 minutes before bedtime and that there are no electronic devices or televisions within the bedroom. I also ask my patients to block blue light and to use blue light filters on their mobile devices. There are also blue light spectacles available. Consider investing in some indoor circadian lighting, which consists of dimmable LED lights that mirror the typical day by having brighter shades in the day and warmer tones for the afternoon and evening.

Medication

Sometimes there is a role for medication such as zopiclone or muscle relaxants like diazepam, but in the long run medications disrupt sleep patterns more and therefore are not recommended (see page 201).

SET YOUR SLEEP GOALS

Now that you have done the sleep assessment on page 186 and have read through the chapter, write down two small things you could do to improve your natural sleep. These can be in the field of exercise, diet and/or mind–body techniques.

The purpose is to do an activity, even if it is for two minutes. If it is easy to do and you can complete it then your nervous system starts to build a new network and learn, thus taking the first steps to a pain-free mindset.

We have now seen how sleep can play a powerful and important role in making your pain worse and that optimising sleep using various techniques can also improve your pain, and even reduce your need for medication, as it did for Sean. As we've seen, an important step in promoting sleep is the role of physical activity and this is what we will look at in the next chapter.

Summary

- There are many significant ways in which sleep loss or deficit can independently cause harm.
- Pain and sleep are bidirectional and they influence each other.
- Improving sleep can reduce the intensity of chronic pain.
- There are both drug and non-drug strategies to achieve an improvement in sleep.
- Most sleep and pain medications disrupt various wave patterns in the sleep cycles and are not suitable for long-term use.
- Mind–body interventions hold great promise for managing pain.

CHAPTER 8

Exercise and Movement

Movement offers us pleasure, identity, belonging and hope. It puts us in places that are good for us.
Kelly McGonigal, Stanford University
psychologist and author

WITHIN PAIN MANAGEMENT, our attitudes towards exercise and movement have changed dramatically in the last decade.

Louise (who we met on page 43) suffers with multiple pain problems including osteoarthritis and fibromyalgia. Until 2017, she was in considerable pain and could do 'fewer than forty steps a day' because of her pain. She was on multiple medications, including high doses of nerve pain tablets and morphine. She had put on considerable weight and this reduced her mobility even further.

This had been gradually worsening and, by 2015, she was mentally very low with profound anxiety and was not keen to socially engage, nor was she comfortable in group settings or on hospital visits: 'I was so overweight by the time I went into hospital. I was 25 stone despite trying to keep weight off. I wasn't eating a lot because I wasn't sleeping and I wasn't active and on those drugs.'

Following two urgent admissions and general anaesthetics for opioid-related constipation and abdominal pain, she was advised to come off the drugs. In order to expend some energy, she was told to 'pace the ward as that would fire the endorphins'.

'That really resonated with me,' she explained to me. 'I put my earphones on and went up and down the ward and I kept that going for days and nights. It really worked and helped. When I got home, if things started to get difficult, I would dance around the living room because it gave me the same effect.'

With the support of her partner, Louise took up hiking, initially on flat paths for short distances with frequent stops. Louise's diagnosis has not changed, but by combining the power of movement and walking with mindfulness-based approaches to sleep and other treatment options, she has been able to come off all her pain medication and has been drug-free for the last three years. Now she is able to walk with no aids, her arthritis is much better, she has lost eight-and-a-half stone and, on most days, she hikes three to five miles a day.

Old versus New Beliefs

For a long time, a standard suggestion for chronic pain patients was rest and inactivity to prevent a flare-up of pain. Now, lots of national and international guidelines promote physical activity and exercise-based movement as an important part of the treatment plan for chronic pain. Movement and exercise can do wonders for chronic pain and, when combined with the other elements of the pain-free mindset approach, will result in significantly improved quality of life and well-being.

Experiments have shown that when we restrict patients from their usual activity and exercise, they become more anxious, tired, depressed and with an increase in pain. When such patients were asked to reduce their daily step count, 88 per cent became more depressed. In fact, a 31 per cent decline in life satisfaction happened when certain subjects were asked to stop exercising for one week.[1]

However, even though national guidelines for conditions like osteoarthritis now strongly recommend movement and exercise, and there are obvious benefits, I still see patients in my pain clinic who tell me that they were advised by a healthcare professional in the near past against doing any form of activity to avoid flare-ups.

Healthcare professionals again tend to focus on the biomedical thought process about structure and healing, which has meant that exercise prescriptions have been closely linked to whether a structure was healing or not. The good news is that some revolutionary new ideas around movement and exercise are now becoming accepted. If we look at it from an evolutionary standpoint, you will understand why, now more than ever, movement can be a powerful force for improving your pain.

I know each one of you might have a different pain and, in your previous interactions with various clinicians, you would have heard talk about core muscles and other specific muscle group exercises. Trying to suggest common exercises for each group is never going to be possible within this book. In fact, researchers at the world-famous Cochrane Collaboration looked at 381 studies of almost 37,000 participants with a wide variety of pain conditions and noted that, while physical activity and exercise did not cause harm, there was so much variety that they could not make definite recommendations regarding one particular kind of exercise.[2]

I also don't believe in the concept that exercise should be done only in a fixed set of repetitions or in a gym with trainers. I know that many of my patients want the reassurance initially of doing it with support and supervision. However, I also know a lot of patients who have some deep worries about exercise and, if their first episode at the gym does not go well, they are put off from any further movement.

Instead, what I am going to suggest is that, once you understand that nociception is not the same as pain (see page 20), you will have the confidence to move without worrying that you are harming yourself. A highly effective way to address pain is not necessarily doing the kind of fitness programmes or repetitions that you see in a gym, but to use movement and exercise as a way of engaging gradually in more activities of daily living and doing activities that you want to do. Such activities may need to be taught and sometimes broken down into their component parts in order to give you the confidence to do them safely.

EXERCISE VERSUS PHYSICAL ACTIVITY

Strictly speaking, physical activity refers to any movement of the skeletal muscles of the body to get somewhere, and exercise often refers to a subcategory of physical activity where you do a predefined set of activities aimed at an end goal. In this chapter I will use these terms interchangeably.

The Importance of Exercise for Persistent Pain

Physical inactivity is the fourth biggest cause of poor health and is responsible for over 5 million deaths a year worldwide.[3] It impacts on all domains and outcomes for people as well as the communities they live in. In fact, it has been called a global health problem by the WHO with one-third of the world's population being physically inactive.[4]

Physical inactivity is said to be responsible for as much as one out of every six deaths and that is the same as being a smoker. Forty per cent of long-term conditions could be prevented if everyone did the daily recommendations for physical activity. The Moving Medicine website is a big collaboration between a number of very important organisations and they have noted that 27 per cent of the population would be considered inactive, meaning that they do not do even 30 minutes of moderate physical activity a week. Up to 33 per cent of children do less than the recommended activity for their age.[5]

As we saw at the beginning of the chapter, for most people, extending their range of motion and carrying out strengthening and aerobic conditioning exercises is not only safe, but necessary to reduce pain.

Exercise can help pain by:

- regulating sleep
- reducing inflammation
- influencing mood and mental health
- combating tiredness and improving your energy levels, thus reducing your perception of pain

215

Exercise is now quite far-reaching in terms of its benefit on the human body:

Building muscle can reduce pain

This muscle-building aspect of exercise has a double advantage:

1. It improves the bulk of muscles and more mitochondria (energy generators).
2. It allows for the muscle to release various chemicals that can reduce pain.

Muscle is the largest consumer of glucose and therefore having more muscle mass to remove this glucose at regular intervals reduces the risk of excess glucose-related inflammation in patients. With physical inactivity, there is a decline in the function of the mitochondria. While mitochondria are found in all cells of the body, they are present in particularly high concentrations in muscle and are increased with physical activity. Inactivity leads to their poor function and can contribute to fatigue and muscle pain.

Myokines

More than anything, the biggest benefit of building muscle through regular physical activity is also a better control of the signalling molecules that are released from the muscle. These are small protein molecules (peptides) called myokines and were discovered in 2000 by Bente Pedersen, an exercise physiologist in Copenhagen.[6] These molecules, which are released on physical activity, not only regulate the muscle but also help with the growth, nutrition and reduction of inflammation and the immune system, thus potentially reducing pain.[7]

Myokines are thought to control the inflammatory chemicals that get produced from fat cells, especially those that are present in and around the intestines of people causing a different kind of obesity called 'TOFI' (thin outside but fat inside). You may think that because you look thin, you don't need to do any physical activity, but if you have abdominal fat (which is the fat that is present inside around the organs) in larger quantities (an apple-type body – see box below), then physical inactivity combined with inflammatory chemicals from your fat cells can put you at higher risk of not just chronic pain but also metabolic conditions like type 2 diabetes.

ARE YOU AN APPLE OR A PEAR?

This is a quick exercise to see whether you are an apple or a pear.

Measure your waist in inches (measure one inch above your belly button) and then your hips in inches (measure the widest part of your bottom, which is the buttocks for some people and the thighs for others).

The ratio of the waist to hip measurement is your apple/pear score. For women, if your score is 0.8 or less, you are a pear and therefore have a lower amount of abdominal fat; if it exceeds 0.8, you are an apple. For men, if your score is 0.9 or less, you are a pear; if it exceeds 0.9, you are an apple.

Exercise slows the ageing process

As the population ages, arthritis and a loss of muscle mass (called sarcopenia) can both cause chronic pain. Ageing also brings on an inflammatory process – known as 'inflammaging' – which contributes to the stress response and can further worsen pain.[8]

Maintaining a healthy lifestyle can be difficult as we age, but it is a critical component for optimising health and improving happiness. Exercise has been shown in numerous studies to impact and sometimes reduce the effect of the ageing process.[9] Older individuals who exercise quite regularly have better balance with improved flexibility and mobility with better control of their blood pressure and/or heart rate.

Physical activity definitely reduces the onset of serious health conditions and a good exercise regime could potentially increase life span by another five years. Ageing does not necessarily lead to frailty and exercise helps us live healthier and longer.[10] By failing to move, you risk amplifying all the problems of chronic pain and simple physical activity can change that.

Exercise increases brain size/function

Some of the biggest advances in our understanding of exercise have, not surprisingly, come from neuroscientists studying the brain and the effect of exercise on the brain.

Seen over 5 million times, neuroscientist Wendy Suzuki claims in her TED Talk that exercise was so transformative that she switched her whole field of research to understand what exercise does to the brain.[11]

'Even a single brief workout can increase the amount of dopamine and other mood-related chemicals immediately,' she says, and it apparently increases our ability to become more focused and attentive and improves reaction times. If we can then change the kind of exercise/movement we do and add in some aerobic exercise then that change can be made to last. Imagine the effect on your mood and pain!

Exercise improves the blood flow and increases the size of certain brain regions like the prefrontal cortex (your rational decision-making area) and the hippocampus (your memory storage place). This increase in your brain ability and more dopamine is advantageous in the short term for your daily function, and can all work to improve mood and more thoughtful decision-making.

All of these changes can help in dampening chronic pain and can occur with the minimum standard open aerobic activity that increases heart rate – three to four times a week, thirty minutes each time.

The runner's high

The well-known runner's high, which clinical psychologist and author Kelly McGonigal calls the 'persistence high', is now understood to be due to an activation of the endocannabinoid system.[12] In fact, for all practical purposes the runner's high is essentially a 'weed hit'.

McGonigal explains in her book *The Joy of Movement* that it's not the physical action of running, but the intensity that we are able to maintain with any activity that brings on that high. She gives an example of a patient who can use exercise as a way of keeping away from pain medications – the daily sessions with the challenges give her the necessary stimulus to keep going.

McGonigal's advice: *Do not too get bogged down by a specific kind of physical activity. Instead, go for an activity that you love. Do it at a moderate intensity for at least 20 minutes.* That is enough to give you the persistence high, which then does wonders for your mental health and pain.

Since the endocannabinoid system provides the balance between the sympathetic nervous system's fight and flight response and the parasympathetic system's rest and digest response, it has multiple effects on different organ systems and can help in pain control as well. Its activation can reduce anxiety and improve social bonding and communication. It rewards both the body and the brain.

> An exercise/physical activity regime of 30 minutes/day can be equal to taking a benzodiazepine drug like diazepam but without any of the side effects.

Mental health disorders, pain and exercise

Exercise can not only relieve anxiety and depression but it leaves people more satisfied and rewarded. Given the massive overlap between pain, anxiety and depression, imagine how much of the pain can be reduced by reducing the anxiety and depression networks using exercise. In fact, a recent review has shown that when exercise is added to antidepressant treatment there are much larger improvements noted than with just medication alone.[13]

Physical activity acts on the same parts of the reward pathway as we saw in Chapter 3 (see page 72), though it is obviously a more socially acceptable solution than illicit drugs. In its extreme, people can get addicted to physical activity and exercise (so-called 'exercise addiction'). However, there is a difference between exercise-related addiction and illicit drug addiction in terms of how it affects the reward pathway. Normally when you are addicted, you experience a high, but after a while, as the nerve circuits get more tolerant, you never experience that high or it becomes more and more short-lived. Like in the case of opioids, you need to keep taking more. With movement and exercise, that tolerance effect doesn't seem to happen and therefore benefits seem to last, though this is still being debated.

The role of the sympathetic nervous system

If you have a continuous overactivity of the sympathetic nervous system, that can be harmful. This can happen if you suffer from anxiety and/or depression. Since the natural response of the nervous system is going to be one of fight, flight or fright and freeze, it can worsen any pre-existing pain.

If your body adopts this state on a continuous basis, it is going to constantly keep giving instructions to the muscles of both your upper and lower back to stay tight and ready to fight the enemy, run away or just freeze and play dead. None of these is useful or advantageous to the muscles. But the nervous system doesn't know this – it is enacting an automatic self-protection mechanism.

This kind of tightness means that the muscle fibres stay locked all the time and the lactic acid builds up in the muscle, activating another substance called 'substance P', which irritates the nerves and can create nociception. This makes the signals feel even worse. When this happens, the brain says, 'I feel more signals coming' and begins to tighten up the muscles even more, hence making this a vicious cycle.

This vicious cycle of tightness and increased tension can be broken by doing only one thing – movement. Movement interrupts the pain cycle and the signals that are being sent telling the body to fight, flight or fright/freeze.

At this point, your pain is a protective (or overprotective) prediction that your central nervous system makes. Pain is often the outcome of the brain's decision to protect you, which could be due to multiple factors out of which tissue injury is only one. So while you would be experiencing pain, there is unlikely to be any harm.

What is important is that you move. It's not important if you work out your upper body or your lower body. It does not matter if you strengthen your core or tone up your muscles. Your muscles are not weak from your specific pain issues – it's more likely they are not functioning efficiently because your pain has stopped you from wanting to move at all.

Trying to keep a level of active movement helps to calm the nerves down over time. Each time you move and they learn that things haven't got worse, you could be building a new pain-free network that will replace the one that has been sending the 'pain' signals. The brain is able to use this principle of neuroplasticity that exercise gives and harness that benefit to improve pain. This is the main reason why exercise is now being suggested for most pain conditions.

THE BENEFITS OF EXERCISE FOR PAIN

The beneficial effect of exercise spans multiple organ systems:

1. Weight loss: physical activity-induced weight loss can reduce pain in some patients.
2. Immune system support: physical activity also fires up the immune system from the brain to the energy systems (mitochondria) within individual cells, thus reducing inflammation.
3. Improved brain function: the improvement in brain capacity and function can help in regulating mood and pain better.
4. Slows down the ageing process and associated inflammation in the body.
5. Increased social connection: exercise when done in groups has a powerful social advantage, and the resulting joy and connection can be pain-relieving.
6. Neuroplasticity: the endorphin rush that comes with exercise helps in moulding and shaping the brain and builds new circuits that can protect against pain.
7. Protects the brain by reducing the amount of inflammatory chemicals produced.
8. Stress resilience: with exercise, the myokines influence the brain and make it more resilient to stress.

Developing an Exercise Mindset

There are generally three ways to view physical activity, as shown in the table overleaf.[14]

Moderate activity	Activities that raise your heart rate or make you breathe faster or feel warmer – you can talk but not sing. Such activities include brisk walking, water aerobics, dancing, doubles tennis, pushing a lawn mower or hiking.
Vigorous activity	Activities that make you breathe hard and fast – you should not be able to say more than a few words without pausing for breath. 75 minutes of vigorous activity can give the same as 150 minutes of moderate activity, and even moderate activities can become vigorous if the activity intensity is increased. Such activities include jogging or running, swimming, riding a bike, walking up the stairs, sports like football, skipping rope, gymnastics and martial arts.
Very vigorous activity	Activities that are performed in short bursts of intense effort and then broken or spaced by periods of rest. These are also known as high-intensity interval training (HIIT). Such activities include lifting heavy weights, circuit training, sprinting up hills, interval running or running up stairs, and doing spin classes.

At this point, with your pain, what are you able to do? Which category would you fit into? (Don't worry if your pain has been so severe that you are not able to fit into any of these categories.)

How physically active are you?

There are multiple exercise programmes that you might have tried and you may have seen various movement specialists like a physiotherapist, osteopath or chiropractor. The questions below are a good starting point to assess your present fitness:

How many days a week can you do a moderate physical activity like a brisk walk?

☐ <2 days ☐ 2–5 days ☐ >5 days

On average, for how many minutes per day do you do that physical activity?

☐ <10 minutes ☐ 10–30 minutes ☐ >30 minutes

How many days a week can you do any strength or resistance exercises for your muscles?

☐ Rarely ☐ 1–3 days ☐ >3 days

With most types of chronic pain, we would still want people to be functionally active and be able to do at least 30 minutes of moderate activity on 5 days of the week with resistance exercises on 3 of them. If your pain prevents you from doing that right now, then see where you find yourself by keeping a diary for the next 7 days, logging your physical activity.

FORMS OF EXERCISE

Broadly, exercises can be:

- **Stretching:** helps to increase flexibility, loosen stiff muscles and improve your range of motion. Stretching is required in both warm-up and cool-down.
- **Strengthening:** tends to focus more on building tone and strength in selected muscle groups.

- **Cardiovascular/aerobic:** these exercises are more generalised like walking, swimming, hiking and bike riding.
- **Balance:** as age increases, exercises to improve balance, gait and agility are increasingly important as they reduce the risk of falls and associated pain.

What kind of beliefs do you hold regarding physical activity and exercise?

- Do you see exercise as something that can be done only when you are pain-free?
- Do you see exercise as something that is done only by healthy people in fancy gyms with lots of equipment and trainers?
- Do you think that it can be a logical choice for patients who are in persistent pain but it may not apply for your situation?

If you answered 'Yes' to all three of these questions then I would suggest that we need to explore that in more detail.

These are important questions that need to be clarified as they will reflect deeply held beliefs that will influence your behaviours regarding any exercise regime that you have.

Where do such beliefs come from?

- You may have been told by someone you trust (your GP, physiotherapist or consultant). Maybe they led you to believe that your pain is due to a structure being 'bone on bone' or that you must not lift certain weights or do certain things until it is fixed. Now that you know that structure has no correlation to pain, can you question that belief that you hold? Because what you are holding is a powerful belief (a nocebo), but nevertheless it is a false belief.

- A consequence of an earlier attempt to do a particular exercise that didn't go well. It may be that you have not been supported in the right manner or you overdid the particular routine based on the understanding you were given. That may have put you off ever trying it again.

Both of these can be powerful barriers to you doing any programme, so think about this and see if they could apply to you.[15] See if you can question those beliefs.

You may be in a place that Stanford psychology professor Carol Dweck calls the 'fixed mindset', where you feel that it won't work or will make your pain worse, so why try it at all.[16] The opposite to the fixed mindset is the 'growth mindset', where setbacks are viewed as opportunities to try something a little differently and go through the process knowing that it will get better. If this is chronic pain with not much nociception, then adopting the exercise mindset will be hugely advantageous to you. The pain-free mindset itself is a form of growth mindset.

So, what is the exercise mindset?

- With any new activity, we have to be prepared to know and accept that we won't get it right the first few times and small pain flares can occur but there is no harm.
- When that flare occurs, it is important to be kind to oneself at that time but not give up.
- Approach it with the intention of starting low in intensity and quality and going slow, and gradually increasing as

confidence starts to increase. Aim to do short bursts of activity to start with (sometimes as little as 20–30 seconds at a time).

- Once you realise that pain isn't getting worse anymore, as Louise found to be true, beliefs get changed and this results in a new neural network.
- Once the new neural network is formed then you progress very quickly.
- Each of us will be different in this growth mindset. As an analogy, it is very much like learning to drive a car. You might be one of those lucky ones who gets it right very quickly. I took my time and needed about 20 lessons before I could take the test. You may be like me and need a lot more support, but once the network is formed you never really forget it.

Fear avoidance

One of the main concerns for patients is the concept of fear avoidance.[17] Since most people confuse nociception with pain and equal hurt to harm, they end up avoiding or staying away from movement or any exercise that they find painful. Sometimes they stop it altogether and this fear of avoiding movement can sometimes be a bigger issue than the actual condition of the muscles/joints/bones. This cycle of fear avoidance can be broken by exposure therapies, which are increasingly being offered by pain specialist physiotherapists to increase patients' confidence.

One of the therapies that has been introduced in recent times is Peter O'Sullivan's cognitive functional therapy model.[18] O'Sullivan is a noted Australian physiotherapist and pain researcher and his model offers a patient-centred integration of good validation and listening, as well as careful understanding of the patient's expectations and fears. Using the model, therapists work with the patient to address those specific fears of movement and coach them to improve the ability to achieve those movements, which can then give them confidence to move more. These kinds of exposure therapies are becoming more popular and may help you if you are avoiding movement out of fear. They work on the same principle of neuroplasticity where the trusted therapist will work with you to do a previously feared movement safely and get you to repeat it until it becomes safe.

Starting to Exercise When in Pain

The NHS website documents that adults should do some form of physical activity daily and recommends strengthening or moderate-intensity activities with weekly targets that are individually tailored.[19] It talks about pacing and gradual increase in intensity, especially if you have been inactive. In my opinion, things are a bit different when someone is in pain.

Hurt does not equal harm

The first step is to accept that hurt will not equal harm. This could mean having a chat with your GP or your specialist physiotherapist or doctor and making sure that the scans or any imaging are well understood, and that you know what changes are due to age and whether there is any risk of injury.

Obviously, I wouldn't expect you to go straight to an intense fitness regime if you haven't done anything in a while. You could speak to your physiotherapist, manual therapist or healthcare professional who understands the concepts in this book to suggest a starting point and help you create a programme:

- Start by defining what exercise/physical activity means to you.
- Don't make any workouts too prescriptive.
- Make sure that whatever exercise you do or plan to do is familiar enough to be safe for you. You don't want to start with a routine you have never done before without supervision.

Start low, go slow

Start with something very simple and easy to do that gives you confidence. You are essentially trying to break an overprotective habit that the brain has got into and teach it a safe new habit.

One technique is to imagine your pain on a scale and, if your levels increase by more than two points from when you started, that could serve as a natural stop. In the beginning when there is an element of deconditioning as well as anxiety, sometimes even the thought of doing certain activities can worsen pain and, in that case, the pain scale is less useful. It is, however, a good benchmark when you start any movement exercise.

I suggest to my patients that they try walking for five- to ten-minute periods. Usually that is possible for most patients. I ask them to walk at a speed they are comfortable with to start. If they can do this once a day to begin with, over a period of a week I ask them to increase it to three times a day. This would mean doing at least 30 minutes of activity a day in total.

Develop a good breathing technique

When you are in pain, you are often prone to slipping into shallow and fast breaths if the pain increases. It is important that you learn how to take deep breaths and relaxation techniques that can help to get this aspect right, such as progressive muscular relaxation (see page 248) and even some forms of meditation or yoga (see pages 204 and 250).

Be kind to yourself

It is natural in the modern digital world to compare your fitness regime with others or compare your present life with pain to who you were without the pain. This is where some techniques like CBT or ACT can be useful to learn (see pages 243–4).

Consider joining a group

We all understand how collective exercise, such as group runs, can be uplifting. That sense of empowerment through a joint action is what Kelly McGonigal has called 'we agency'. Joint events and charities all run on that collective spirit of joy, optimism and hope that exercise can bring to the management of mood and eventually pain.

Often doing activities in a group can be liberating and supportive, but it is a fine balance in terms of becoming too competitive. It is important to do what you can do comfortably.

Keep a log

Use an online tracker or mobile tracker of your activity. This will offer the dual advantage of seeing trends and gradual improvement and, at the same time, can help you to notice a pattern when some days are more difficult.

Anticipate flare-ups and plan

You can minimise setbacks by starting small, but at some point a flare-up will happen. Have a plan of action to overcome that and then start again. The ultimate aim with movement is to be able to try to do all movements without the pain getting worse. If you have been in pain for a long time, you will have formed some unwanted and overprotective networks and neurotags that have to be undone with time (see page 116). Initially these neurotags will increase the perception of 'pain' and cause a flare-up.

Consider adding music

To improve motivation to exercise or move, consider adding in a 'power song' to enhance the new neural network that will form. McGonigal suggests that a power song should inspire, have a strong beat (120–140bpm), an energetic feel and matching lyrics, and meaning to you.[20] This is because music can reduce the perceived effort and can make exercise more enjoyable and easier. The brain is hardwired to hear music as an invitation to move. Music can channel and reawaken old nerve circuits and lay down fresh ones.

Any movement will do

With the new science around the role of muscle, exercise and the myokines (see page 216), I can't recommend one particular form of exercise over another, but instead it needs to be a combination of therapies – the most important aspect is that you do something that you love, are comfortable doing and can do safely.

The popular approaches available in the NHS and privately are physiotherapy, Pilates, recreational sports, tai chi, spin classes, yoga, cycling and a myriad of other physical activities. As Bronnie Thompson, physiotherapist and fibromyalgia sufferer, highlights, reasons for doing exercise vary a lot and it can be done in different ways – she argues that the more that activity or exercise is easy to do and can be incorporated into your daily life, the better it is.[21]

Other gentle starting points for those with pain are taking the stairs at your workplace instead of the lift, setting a reminder to ensure that you sit up or move about every 20–25 minutes, or set small exercises to park further and further away from your destination so that you can walk those extra few metres.

Work with a therapist

With the number of false beliefs around exercise and the myriad options available, finding the *right* professional at the *right* place and the *right* time are becoming essential in getting the *right* support for your pain.

Many patients have told me that they have had physiotherapy, or some other allied therapy, in the past with little or marginal improvement. While it has been difficult to get relief in some patients, there's more to exercise and pain than just thinking about core muscle strengthening/bone alignment or muscle and ligament problems, and very few studies have been done that convincingly prove that exercise and core strengthening improve pain and reduce disability.

There is a risk that therapy sessions can become passive if what you are getting is massage, acupuncture or infrared therapy, and it is important that you do the homework that they often give you. This is where things get difficult for many pain patients as they feel confident or are able to do the exercises under supervision, but are not able to do them on their own.

It is therefore important to seek a therapist who is comfortable with the new knowledge in pain and the concepts in this book, and is able to work with you and help you create a programme that reduces danger, improves the perception of safety and offers support and coaching as needed. There are now specialist pain physiotherapists, who are very experienced physiotherapists and are able to help, so please do seek support.

Summary

- Physical inactivity is one of the main causes of long-term sickness and is now considered a global health problem.
- Exercise and physical activity are essential to pain control and improving quality of life.
- Exercise and movement have tremendous benefits affecting every organ system of the body, including mental and physical health, thus benefiting pain control.
- Exercise improves the function of the brain and builds muscle, both of which have a beneficial effect on pain control.
- Flare-ups are common when we start a new physical activity regime while in pain.
- Pain does not equal damage.
- Start low and go slow with your preferred physical activity plan.
- Work with a good therapist/coach if needed.

CHAPTER 9

Therapies of the Mind and Body

Between stimulus and response there is a space. In that space is our power to choose our response. In our response lies our growth and our freedom.

Viktor Frankl, Austrian neurologist,
psychiatrist and Holocaust survivor

I HAVE BEEN looking after Praveen for close to ten years now and I have seen her pain journey. Her referral to me was for management of pelvic pain that had come on after a routine gynaecological operation. Unfortunately, it was complicated by an infection that required a repeat surgery to stitch it up and, at that time, a nerve got trapped. Since then, she has been left with a 'ripping, stabbing, horrible' pain that, over time, had spread to involve her whole body. A few years ago she also got diagnosed with breast cancer and underwent chemotherapy, surgery and radiotherapy, and that further weakened her and caused flare-ups of her pain and fatigue.

A busy solicitor who had got married just two months before her first-ever surgery, she has since then, despite the pain, gone on to have two children, which has given the impetus she needed to go on and look after herself and family. She still has pain but has gained a lot by doing a pain management programme. As she describes, it was an 'ideal jumping board' for her to take charge of her life. Her desire was to become a mother and stay off strong drugs and, to a great extent, she has achieved that. She did have good social support, so it was considerably easier than for someone who may not have those advantages. Nevertheless, it took her almost 18 months to reach that place and there were times when she had occasional bad days and she reached out for some extra help and support from her healthcare professionals.

Once my colleague and I explained to her the nature of chronic neuropathic pain, she understood what her prognosis would be and refocused her attention on the things that mattered the most to her: time with her family, becoming a mother, understanding her limits and keeping active. As she confessed, it wasn't easy but it got better over time. She continued to get support from a psychologist for her mood and changed her whole diet to reduce inflammation. Most importantly, however, exercise and psychological support were some of her mainstays for pain control over the years.

A lot of mind–body techniques, especially those that influence our thinking, are approaches that should be first line and imparted to the patient at the same time as their first medication, scan or physiotherapy session. I am confident that if we could include some of these techniques much earlier with good pain science education then healthcare costs due to overuse of opioid drugs or unnecessary surgery would drop significantly.

TERMINOLOGY

There are lots of names you will come across: complementary, integrative, alternative, CAM, holistic, etc. Traditionally, 'complementary' therapies were often thought of as techniques that are provided alongside conventional medical drugs or interventions, while 'alternative' techniques were thought of as instead of the conventional medicine. Alternative therapies are often an extremely sensitive topic about which people hold very strong opinions and sometimes irrational beliefs.

For the purposes of this chapter, and indeed the pain-free mindset in general, I believe that most of these techniques are now part of mind–body therapies. Some, like reiki and spiritual therapy or homeopathy, have hardly any scientific evidence to back them up, while others like yoga, hypnosis and meditation/mindfulness are mainstream techniques with many studies showing the benefits, but they all work for certain patients.

Mind–Body Therapies

In the old biomedical model, the concept that thoughts and emotions can influence pain was not accepted as scientific enough, so it was never respected. However, as we have seen in previous chapters, the mind and body are connected quite deeply.

This developing field is called psychoneuroimmunology; it examines the way our behaviours and emotions influence our body's nervous and immune systems. It firmly establishes that acute psychological stress acts on the same brain structures as physical trauma and sensitises the nervous, endocrine and immune systems. There is now increasing proof that reducing this stress by using a variety of non-drug techniques can achieve reduction in pain and reduce the need for strong medications like opioids.[1]

They are empowering

Mind–body therapies have the power to promote care that is personalised to you, with higher satisfaction and more control in your hands. Ideally, they treat the whole person and could be learnt by you so that you can practise them at home to maintain the benefits.

Like many treatments in chronic pain, there is a likelihood that the placebo effect is responsible for a big proportion of the benefits. To me, that isn't a problem in itself as they, at least for the most part, aren't harmful as stronger pain medications or surgery can be. While they may not be any more effective than medications or interventions, there will be people for whom these therapies will be transformative. When you combine these with the other elements of the pain-free mindset, the chances of overall pain control are much higher.

One size does not fit all

What we don't know is 'which specific treatment is most effective for which particular patient under what specific condition', and high-quality evidence has been difficult to get.[2] However, this does not mean they don't work; it is just that we need more funding and research to know who they can work on. At the time of writing, researchers have looked at 9,400 patients from 75 studies and noted that CBT can reduce pain and distress.[3] Many therapies vary in what they set out to achieve, but they are broadly united in the sense that they promote healing with very few side effects.

The patient–therapist relationship is key

An especially important but subjective component is how the therapist interacts with you. This is called 'therapeutic alliance' and is sometimes as important as the actual treatment itself.

The earlier the better

While some of these treatments are sought in the first instance, like physiotherapy or osteopathic treatment, often patients enter the biomedical model by going down the route of drugs or interventions. Once everything has been tried and 'conventional' treatments haven't worked, they then get referred to a pain clinic, often after a few years. This is a mistake in my opinion.

Consider the plight of Tina, who we met on page 81. When initial physiotherapy, which was all about biomedical core exercises, didn't help her prolapsed disc, she got referred to a surgeon and had a disc removal surgery, which didn't work. With post-surgical nerve damage pain, she was referred again for physiotherapy and, four years after the injury, finally gained an alliance with an influential physiotherapist. She recollected, 'He took a totally different approach to any of the other physiotherapists. He taught me about the complexity of pain. I started to understand all the different factors that go into the experience of pain. It had never occurred to me that there was a bigger picture.'

That bigger picture has been embraced by most of my patients who have found one or a combination of therapies useful, and maybe even life-changing, with no side effects. At the time of writing, physiotherapy is the only treatment that is offered regularly on the NHS. However, there are reports of some GPs having local arrangements to provide some mind–body therapies via community partners, so speak to your GP and see what is available.

The evidence for any of these working on their own does not exist, but combining it early in your pain journey is going to be the factor that predicts long-term improvement. As Tina recollected, 'If I'd met that physiotherapist within the first six weeks, then I could have made that paradigm shift early on. But I couldn't make a paradigm shift without being taught. Simply because I didn't know.'

PAIN EDUCATION

Knowledge is powerful and understanding the new ways of thinking about pain, like you have read in this book, may itself have some therapeutic effect.

American pain researchers looked at 13 randomised controlled trials and concluded that there was strong evidence that pain neuroscience education can improve knowledge, reduce disability, improve pain ratings, reduce catastrophisation, reduce fear avoidance and behaviours regarding pain, increase physical movement and, more importantly, help to reduce the number of patient visits to GPs or emergency departments.[4]

Understanding your pain therefore reduces anxiety and improves knowledge, and can also help you have a more informed discussion about your treatment choices with the healthcare professionals working with you to overcome your pain.

Relaxation is key

Chronic pain, in some ways, is a form of chronic stress as there is a significant role of the stress hormone cortisol and the overactivity of the sympathetic nervous system in activating the fight and flight response continuously. This stress, as we saw in Chapter 5, activates the immune system of the brain and causes the microglia (the policemen) to go rogue and cause inflammation. This continued stress has an impact on every organ system in the body. Most mind–body therapies will calm down the overactive system and help you relax and reduce pain.

Choosing the Right Therapy for You

The therapies listed below are not exhaustive or complete, nor are they my recommendations, but it should give you a starting point. Many of these, especially CBT-based techniques, are combined and offered within standard NHS pain management programmes and many physiotherapists combine manipulation and heat/massage/acupuncture within their sessions.

Be open to the therapy and treatment and try to establish a good relationship with your therapist. Be very clear about how much it is costing and what benefit it is giving you over a few days to weeks or months.

I recommend that you move, over time, from therapies that are done *for* you, through those that are done *with* you, to those that *you do yourself* with support (so-called 'supported self-management') – see page 268 for more on this. This is the most ideal and cost-effective option.

241

Another way to decide which of these therapies can work for you is this suggestion by doctor and pain sufferer Amy Orr: you could write down the therapies that you want to try and rate them based on:[5]

- short-term benefit: a few days (<1 week)
- long-term benefit: many weeks (> 1 month)
- cost (whether covered by NHS/insurance or self-pay)
- how far you have to travel to get there and the time it takes

---

YOU WILL HAVE TO PAY FOR MOST THERAPIES

Previously, acupuncture, osteopathy and chiropractic therapy and massage were funded by the NHS, but the last official guidance suggested that none of these were cost-effective or beneficial in the long term so they were not funded. Acupuncture has come back in the good books in the most recent draft NICE guidance but who knows how/when that will change?

If you find a therapy that works for you and makes you feel better, then that is what matters. Unfortunately, it then comes down to cost and affordability for you.

Physiotherapy

This is the most common and well-recognised of therapies within the healthcare setting. Physiotherapists are generally considered experts in rehabilitation and are vital to most hospitals and GP practices. Physiotherapists have great experience and skill in managing pain after surgery using good clinical examination skills combined with knowledge of appropriate exercises for various age groups to achieve stretch, strength or control. Many have trained further in acupuncture and even mobilisation techniques for improving joint movement. Much of the advance in pain neuroscience in the last 20 years has come from the work of physiotherapists with a special interest in pain, so there are some physiotherapists who have a very good understanding of the new pain science. The Physiotherapy Pain Association is their umbrella organisation (see Resources, page 312).

Behavioural therapy

This is the most commonly available and well-known set of therapies for holistic management of pain and various mental health conditions. Since there is a considerable overlap between pain and mood, it makes sense to go for therapies that can help with both. As I have said before, if there is no nociception, then pain that is coming from a sensitised nervous system can certainly respond to these therapies, and there will be very few side effects.

Behavioural therapies have a common focus in making people aware of certain behaviours that happen due to thoughts or beliefs, and then helping them change those thoughts, and consequently the behaviours, so they can decrease pain and reduce suffering.

Cognitive behavioural therapy (CBT)

This is the most common form of behavioural therapy. Here your thoughts, feelings, physical sensations and actions are thought of as four ends of a hot cross bun and are often deeply connected. Negative thoughts can reinforce the connections while positive thoughts can lead to changes in the other three areas, leading to practical ways to improve the mind and its ability to react to pain and other stressful situations. The therapist usually tries to gently challenge those negative thoughts and help restructure them with positive options. Sessions usually last for 30–60 minutes and often you can get up to 8–10 sessions either one-to-one or as a group. It can be as effective as other treatments, including medications, especially for pain and mental health issues.

Acceptance and commitment therapy (ACT)

This is an increasingly common form of behavioural therapy and it uses mindfulness and acceptance strategies to increase your psychological flexibility. The objective is not to challenge the difficult or negative thoughts, but to be 'present' and mindful of them and accept them, and then define your desired values and act upon those values rather than trying to change the negativity.

Dialectical behaviour therapy (DBT)

This is another evidence-based psychotherapy approach, initially developed for conditions where there is an emotional regulation issue. It has now been trialled for pain as well and it involves components of mindfulness with acceptance and then change, along with distress tolerance and learning new communication skills.

Compassion-focused therapy (CFT)

This form of therapy integrates self-compassion alongside traditional CBT to promote mental and emotional healing. It brings together some of the findings from neuroscience and evolutionary psychology, such as the threat, drive and soothe systems, to train the mind to experience and develop compassion.

Emotional awareness and expression therapy (EAET)

Another new therapy becoming popular for fibromyalgia treatment, this represents a fusion of other techniques with a focus on pain education, emotional exposure and related therapies, along with techniques like expressive writing and revisualisation to improve outcomes and reduce pain.

Eye movement desensitisation and reprocessing (EMDR)

This form of therapy was originally developed for PTSD and works on the basis that sometimes some forms of pain and other traumatic episodes are stored as maladaptive neural networks. These networks/memories can be desensitised and then processed safely using bilateral eye movements or pulses or tones to relieve the symptoms of trauma.

Cognitive functional therapy (CFT)

This is another holistic physiotherapy-led behavioural therapy that focuses on a strong therapeutic alliance combined with cognitive training/gradual exposure to movement and lifestyle change, all provided in an integrated manner for low back pain and other musculoskeletal pains.

Somatic tracking and somatic experiencing

While somatic tracking is part of the larger concept of somatic experiencing, both are therapies aimed at processing emotional trauma – events that happen suddenly, like an accident, major surgery or a natural disaster – or developmental trauma, as in abuse or neglect while growing up. The aim is to ultimately rewire the sensitised nervous system by observing your body sensations and then reinterpreting them in a safer and productive way.

Mindfulness

Simply put, mindfulness is paying attention to the moment; observing the moment without being influenced by it. It can be practised in a completely non-religious way and has become immensely popular for many conditions including chronic pain. Mindfulness is not the same as meditation. Meditation is one aspect of mindfulness training, but mindfulness is a state of mind. It is a way to apply that process of thinking to various normal events, routines and daily activities. It doesn't need to come with changing your lifestyle, nor is it only for certain groups of people. Often programmes like MBSR (see page 139) have a core component of mindfulness that is combined with movement practice like yoga.

Mindfulness has a few important aspects:

Paying attention

Mindfulness is about trying to change the infrequent and constantly shifting attention that we have. The normal human attention span is quoted as being seven seconds. We want to move to a more purposeful awareness of the task that we are engaged in. It sounds quite an easy thing to do, but in reality can be quite a difficult state to achieve.

Let us think for a moment about how we structure our day. Even starting from a simple meal like breakfast, can you really remember what you ate, how you ate it and what you were doing at that point in time? Mindfulness encourages us to reflect on all these times and reduce the multitasking nature of our lives.

Mindfulness aims to try to stop the pointless chatter that sometimes goes on in our minds about the past and future. This can often be very distracting and counterproductive, fuelling the anxiety or hyper vigilance that will worsen pain. Stress reduction is as important as reducing pain, and this can be achieved with diverse ways such as mindful eating, mindful breathing and mindful meditation.

Sometimes being mindful can make you aware of strong emotional feelings that you may want to deliberately suppress. If this is you, you might need to work with a specialist first to accept and work through such feelings to move forward.

Non-judgemental nature

Mindfulness tries to develop the ability for us to be more curious and compassionate and non-judgemental. This phrase of non-judgement is especially important because it allows us to create a space between what happens to us and how we react to it. This skill becomes useful when pain flare-ups occur.

When you experience a flare-up, it is often an immediate, involuntary, subconscious, automatic response to the occurrence of pain. But if we can learn to take a moment to take a deep breath, be mindful and non-judgemental, that can reduce its intensity.

Acceptance

There are certain points and periods in our life when we can expect to have components of physical and emotional pain, but we have choices we can make on how we decide to deal with it. We can decide the intensity of suffering, and being mindful is to ensure that the event is accepted and the learning is made, so that the pain does not get transmitted, amplified or magnified. This does not necessarily mean accepting the pain, but is about the acceptance of the choices available to you.

BODY SCAN

A body scan is a useful way of using mindfulness practice to alleviate chronic pain. It generally takes about 20–30 minutes and enhances your ability to bring your full attention to your experiences as they happen in the present moment – this is helpful when you are in a pain flare-up or your emotions or thoughts feel out of control. It also trains you to explore and be with pleasant and unpleasant sensations in your body without trying to change anything.

PROGRESSIVE MUSCULAR RELAXATION (PMR)

This is another simple and effective relaxation technique for stress and anxiety management. I often recommend it for my patients and it is an easy technique to practise and learn. The aim is to bring attention to a group of muscles in one area and then tense them for a period of five to ten seconds, before releasing the tension using breathing techniques. It can initially take some practice but can result in a greater amount of relaxation and thus a reduction in pain.

There are a number of free guided body scans and PMR routines online (see also Resources, page 312).

Acupuncture

Acupuncture stems from the Chinese philosophy of energy flowing through channels known as meridians, which lie just below the skin. The energy imbalances in these meridians are used for the diagnosis of disease. Acupuncturists insert very fine needles into the skin to balance energy flow. This needle placement technique takes into consideration the pain location, frequency and duration, as well as intensity.

Traditional Chinese acupuncture is based in the belief that an energy (qi) or 'life force' flows through the body through the meridians. Practitioners who adhere to traditional beliefs believe that when this qi does not flow freely through the body, it can cause illness or pain. Acupuncture is designed to restore the flow of qi and restore health. The Western theory of acupuncture believes that it produces a release of local endorphins (the body's natural painkillers). There are various versions of delivering this – with herbs, electrical stimulation, plasters and patches. They can be done just around the ear and can still give benefit.

Research shows that acupuncture can provide a modest reduction in neck and low back pain and various forms of arthritis. This can improve function and quality of life.[6] Acupuncture calms the emotional centres like the limbic system or the amygdala.[7]

Emotional freedom technique (EFT)

This form of acupuncture, known as 'tapping', uses the fingertips to essentially 'tap' on the same traditional Chinese meridians to 'unblock' the energy points, thus releasing any blocks and relieving pain. This is becoming quite popular, especially in patients who have ongoing anxiety or trauma-related issues.

Yoga and tai chi/qi gong

These practices combine meditation, slow movements, deep breathing and relaxation, and have been found to be helpful in controlling pain.

Yoga originated on the Asian subcontinent and has now massively increased in popularity in the West.[8] A different number of yoga schools (ashtanga/Iyengar/hatha/Bikram/vinyasa) now flourish. They all help in self-development and achieving peace through understanding the mind and body.

Most yoga practices increase muscle tone while incorporating the principles of meditation and relaxation. Make sure to inform the instructor of your condition so they can adjust the different poses and exercises for you. There is an NHS guide that gives a good background to the forms of yoga and the main yoga organisations in the UK (see Resources, page 312).

Tai chi and qi gong are old Chinese movement-based mind–body techniques. Qi gong practice emphasises movement, mind exercises, relaxation and breathing techniques in a less demanding fashion than tai chi. Tai chi is martial-art-like and focuses on the slow and flowing movements from posture to posture. This type of gentle flowing movement:

- relieves stress
- increases flexibility
- improves balance
- promotes a sense of centredness
- promotes well-being

Both qi gong and tai chi provide a good balance between gentle strength building and flexibility.

Chiropractic

Chiropractors are one of the most popular complementary therapists practising in the UK today to help with pain conditions. They are often one of the first groups of healthcare professionals seen by the public when they get a flare-up of their spinal pain.

Chiropractors often focus on the diagnosis and treatment of musculoskeletal or mechanical disorders, and their primary method of treatment is by manipulation or adjustment of the bone structure, thus hoping to relieve pain.

Chiropractors believe that biomechanical and structural changes of the spine can affect the nervous system and manipulation of the spinal area can restore balance, ease pressure on the nerve and improve health.

Their biomechanical view has been at odds with how we view nociception and pain. Their emphasis often on structural alignment creates a nocebo effect amongst patients and can affect them adversely. These days, chiropractors are becoming aware of the possible damage they may be causing by such a narrative and are changing the way they communicate.

Osteopathy

Like chiropractic, osteopathy generally focuses on the assumption that fascia – our connective tissue – can become shortened or tethered, which can often start or amplify pain. Using various manipulation techniques and combinations of massage and mobilisation, osteopaths help provide pain relief by improving alignment and regulating blood flow. Osteopathy can be learnt by many healthcare professionals and is regulated by the General Osteopathic Council in the UK. They are often one of the first healthcare professionals that patients in pain see. Cranial osteopathy is a more gentle mix of osteopathy and chiropractic massage focusing primarily at the base of the skull, desensitising the nerves in that area.

Biofeedback

Biofeedback is the technique of using our body's biological signals to inform us about the state of our body and then using that information to make changes to our breathing and heart rate using various techniques.[9] Strictly speaking, biofeedback is a form of training rather than treatment, so after a certain period, learning to self-regulate is key.

The information can be obtained by measuring a patient's heart rate, breathing, muscle tension, the amount of sweat on the skin, blood pressure, skin temperature and even brainwaves. Once this information is obtained, feedback is provided to the patient and various cognitive/mental exercises and breathing techniques are then taught, which enable them to influence those measurements towards a desired 'normal'. We would normally think that these signals are beyond our control, but biofeedback helps us understand that we have more power than we know.

Biofeedback is extremely useful in managing the stress associated with conditions like migraine, jaw pain and fibromyalgia. A study on chronic back pain showed that biofeedback alone can improve pain relief and reduce muscle tension and depression.[10] Biofeedback can be combined with other therapies to enhance overall pain relief. Examples of biofeedback include heart rate variability testing (HRV). Biofeedback devices are available either via qualified therapists or sometimes for personal use incorporated into your phone or other dedicated wearable device. One thing to remember is that most wearables are much more reliable when you use them to understand a trend rather than one-off measurements.

Hydrotherapy

This involves the use of water at various temperatures and it covers a number of water-based techniques like water massage, mineral baths, cold water plunges and hot tubs/ Jacuzzis, or water-based exercises where gravity can be eliminated/reduced.

The main purpose is to use either hot or cold water to change temperature-based regulatory mechanisms and thereby influence pain perception and, in some cases, facilitate muscle relaxation.

Hypnosis

Hypnosis is becoming quite popular in mainstream medical health. There is increasing use of some of its aspects around communication and language in preoperative reduction of patient anxiety. There is some evidence for its use in acute and chronic pain.[11]

Hypnosis works by altering the processing of pain and other sensory signals in the spinal cord and the brain, and reduces the perception of these signals in various other parts of the brain. It also decreases the emotional response, especially in a region called the anterior cingulate cortex. Hypnotic analgesia has been used for managing pain that comes from childbirth, surgeries, burn dressing, low back pain and headaches, and some chronic pain conditions like IBS and cancer pain.

Hypnosis involves taking patients into a trance-like state. In scientific terms, this involves making the brain more malleable to new learning during the critical phase of suggestion. It is during this phase that the therapist can make meaningful changes to pain perception and intensity. Lots of good hypnotherapists then teach patients self-hypnosis, which can make it more sustainable. Hypnotherapy has great potential in also treating mental health issues around deep-seated trauma and its manifestation, which may on the surface seem harmful but for the brain would be part of its desire to protect.

Myofascial therapy

This form of touch and stretch therapy is particularly focused on mobilising the myofascial plane, which is essentially the combined muscles and connective tissue of the body that lines the muscles called the fascia. Myofascial pain is one of the commonest conditions I see with patients in pain. In this condition, multiple trigger points or tight bands can be felt in various body muscles. These shortened muscles and trigger points can then irritate adjoining nerves, bones and joints, thus amplifying the pain.[12] Lengthening the muscle, trigger point manipulation and injections can all help aided by further physiotherapy.

Dry needling and intramuscular stimulation (IMS)

These are a variation of acupuncture where the injections and needles are placed in various muscle groups, but not part of the acupuncture Chinese point system. Unlike acupuncture, where needles when placed at specific points then stay there for the session, in IMS, they are removed within a few seconds of application. There are many theories of IMS and a popular form is called the 'Gunn IMS', named after Chan Gunn, the Canadian researcher.[13] He suggested that muscle hypersensitivity can happen with ageing underlying bones and that these tight short muscles can be made to lengthen easing pain.

Journaling/expressive writing

Journaling is as simple as keeping a gratitude journal and writing for 15–20 minutes every day about something that went well in your day and with regards to your pain.

At a neuroscientific level, it seems that the physical action of doing the writing alters and changes the nerve circuits to fire differently. When you have the ability to put your thoughts regarding pain and how it makes you feel to paper, it makes a difference in how your brain understands your pain and creates a narrative, which can separate you from the pain.

Keep in mind that you do not have to share your writing with anyone. Write to and for yourself, and if that makes you uncomfortable, simply address your writing to 'dear friend' and just go on to say how your pain is making you feel today:

- What did the pain prevent you from doing that was important to you?
- What have you done to stop the pain?

- Did it help or make the pain feel worse?
- Has the pain been holding in one place or has it been moving and where to?
- Is it causing you frustration or anger?
- Do you feel at peace with your pain today?

A concept developed by social psychologist James Pennebaker, expressive writing can have a benefit on your immune system and improve mental health. Though the effects are short-lived, they are very useful and, most importantly, free.[14]

Aromatherapy

Chronic pain can often be an intensely emotional experience. While the connection between pain and other emotions and sensations is still being researched, the sense of smell has certainly been anecdotally found to be useful. We know that certain smells can remind us of painful or pleasant memories. There are other smells that can bring on nausea or strong aversion.

Aromatherapy refers to the use of highly concentrated essential oils from plants and other sources to reduce anxiety and manage stress and thereby improve pain. Oils such as lavender, peppermint and chamomile are produced from the plant sources by a process of distillation to produce the oils, which are then either inhaled or rubbed on to the skin. When inhaled, studies show their benefit for kidney pain and children's pain. Topical application has been found to help with low back, neck and knee pain.[15]

The reasons for its benefit are still being researched. One possibility is that the molecules of the oil when inhaled are preferentially affecting the amygdala and other structures of the brain, thus distracting the brain from the pain. Paul

Christo, pain physician at Johns Hopkins University, states that peppermint, clove, eucalyptus and German chamomile all have good pain-relieving properties with no side effects.[16] While eucalyptus can be good for inflammatory pain, clove is better for nerve pain. Rose, fennel, balsam fir and chamomile are good for bone pain.

Certified medical aromatherapists are able to help advise and prescribe appropriate aromatherapy solutions and can help you decide on the right route of application. In recent years, ultrasonic diffusers and vaporisers present new methods of aerosolisation and oil delivery.

Music therapy

We have already seen the role of the power song to help with exercise (see page 232). Music has been used for thousands of years to change mood and reframe emotions. It has been shown to reduce anxiety and pain/stress and calm the sympathetic nervous system, and offers a safer way to let out the stress chemicals.

Music therapy refers to the hearing of music, the act of singing or playing an instrument. It is safe and easy to offer and evidence is growing steadily for its use in conditions like low back pain, arthritis and cancer, as well as acute postoperative pain.[17] The compositions of Tim Janis, for example, are now played in many healthcare settings. The soothing music at a slower pace of 60–80bpm reduces muscle tension and eases pain.

Energy and biofield therapies

Energy or touch healing are traditionally Far Eastern and South Asian cultural philosophies that are now gaining presence in the West. While there is healthy scepticism, there is also biological plausibility. After all, we do accept that electrical currents are being generated in our body and that this movement of current does generate some changes in and around our cells. We don't have the technology to measure that force, but the assumption is that it is possible to feel and change that. Energy healing takes that assumption that every living creature generates a bioenergy field that can be altered by trained practitioners to modify or change and thus restore balance, and in the process reduce pain or anxiety and stress.

Energy healing can be done with contact or even non-contact with the practitioner using a non-touch technique. Examples of such healing techniques include chakra healing, crystal healing and Jin Shin Jyutsu.[18]

Touch therapy

Touch is an integral aspect of human development and is known to calm the autonomic nervous system. It can be delivered by both humans and other creatures. Even earthing or grounding could be considered a form of touch therapy. Grounding works on the principle that our ancestors would use ground contact as a way of reducing the build-up of oxidative stress by exchanging electric current with the earth – a known storehouse of electrons. An example of a therapist-delivered touch therapy is reiki. Another form of touch- and pressure-based treatment is neuromuscular therapy developed by Dr Stanley Lief in the thirties.

A typical example of animal-delivered touch is equine-assisted therapy.[19] One of my patients – Lucy – helps out at a horse farm partly because working with horses and touching them gives her calm and reduces her pain. Animal-assisted therapy is a huge umbrella term for a wide variety of activities that are done to help with a patient's physical and mental health (animals can include horses, dogs, cats, pigs and birds), and this involves the energy and touch as well.

Massage therapy

A therapeutic massage is performed by many healthcare professionals and massage therapists. A variation of the massage technique using Chinese principles forms the philosophy behind reflexology as well. Massage broadly involves soft tissue manipulation to alleviate pain, leading to restoration of health and well-being.[20] A lot of my patients go for a massage therapy session on a fortnightly to monthly basis.

Massage therapy sessions can be divided into four approaches:

1. *Gentle body work*, which is craniosacral osteopathy or Swedish massage. These techniques increase body relaxation and a restoration of a state of equilibrium. Gentle body work techniques are usually best suited for pain management, at least in the initial phase, as any more rigorous techniques generally tend to worsen the pain.
2. *Structural body work* of which examples are Rolfing. This kind of body work tries to alter the structure by bringing about a change in the soft tissue architecture of the body, such as the muscles or ligaments, and possibly even the tendons. These can in the short term worsen the pain before improving it.
3. *Deep tissue body work*, such as neuromuscular therapy, deep tissue massage and myofascial release. These are generally done for the alleviation of pain and discomfort.

4. *Movement therapy or re-education*. Examples include the Feldenkrais Method, the Alexander technique, the Gokhale Method and the Rolf Movement. These therapies vary in the amount of hands-on work and they aim to alter a person's habit rather than cause any physical change. The change in the body posture often reduces muscle strain and tension in various parts of the body and that can also help maintain the results of structural body work.

A few studies have explored the role of massage generally for pain management. Most conclude that individual techniques by themselves do not give much benefit, but when massage can be combined with other exercises and education, the benefits definitely outweigh standalone treatments. A study from 2015 looking into massage therapy for fibromyalgia was quite optimistic and noted that it resulted in large reductions in pain and also improvement in anxiety and depression.[21]

Ayurveda

Ayurveda is an old Indian system of traditional and alternative medicine that is combined with a different set of beliefs about the human body that governs the entire prescription range of medication and herbs. It is based on the principle that everything is connected – for example, mind, body and spirit – and that everyone is made of five basic elements: space, air, fire, water and earth. These combine to form three life forces or energies, called doshas. Sickness is an imbalance between these three forces and herbal medicines are given alongside natural remedies and lifestyle recommendations to ease pain and improve health. It essentially treats the person as a whole and is also being researched as an add-on for pain management.[22]

Homeopathy

Based on the principle of like cures like, this is a highly criticised alternative therapy that seems to be still very popular in many parts of Europe and Asia. It is based on the notion that substances that can cause illness in healthy people can also cure those symptoms in sick people when given at very low dilutions. Multiple scientific appraisals have shown that the quality of evidence is very low and any benefit seems to be very difficult to separate from the placebo effect.[23] The actual substances provided as homeopathic medicine are naturally occurring plant and animal extracts, diluted with water sometimes as much as 30 times.

Naturopathy

This form of healing is very holistic and has been present for centuries. Naturopaths mainly are well-versed in using natural therapies and treatments such as fasting, nutrition, water intake and exercise. They also incorporate other alternative therapies such as homeopathy, acupuncture and herbal medicine, as well as newer modalities. The philosophy assumes that if provided with natural support then the body can heal itself.

Orthotic aids and other physical therapies

While these are not mind–body techniques in themselves, many therapists use a lot of these devices and adjuncts as part of their other therapies so they can aid in the whole process.

Splints, taping and casts are often provided by specialists to help with various painful conditions either before or after surgery, sometimes even when surgery is not needed. Taping can be a good alternative to splinting as it is more flexible and allows for greater movement. Other forms of orthotic adjustments can be done for pelvic tilt and limb shortening, and they can help on a personalised basis when needed.

Other physical therapies that are often used by many of these professionals as part of their treatment plan include:

1. *Low-level laser therapy*: good-quality, low-level light lasers have had some benefit in reducing pain, but it is rarely offered these days due to lack of awareness.

2. *Magnet therapies*: these again have waves of popularity and can help as a form of energy healing.

3. *Transcutaneous electrical nerve stimulation (TENS):* a very economical and easy-to-use technique, this is often used by acute pain teams in hospitals and also recommended for use in chronic pain management. It works by improving local blood flow and blocking some of the 'gates' in the spinal cord that send signals to the brain from the area of 'pain'. You can adjust the frequency and wavelength to your need.

4. *Ultrasound therapy*: physiotherapists often add in ultrasonic waves as they can help in increasing blood flow and accelerate healing to help with some patients.

5. *Shock wave therapy*: this is increasingly common in non-scientific literature. The theory behind it is that areas of poor healing pain can persist, and shock waves target these areas and agitate them, inducing inflammation and activating the body's immune system to complete the job.

We've now seen more than 30 different mind–body techniques that have been shown to be very useful in overcoming pain and can be as effective as and sometimes more successful than traditional medicine or surgery. The scientific evidence for these techniques is increasing and I would encourage you to read more about them and try them out to see which ones can be added to your pain-free mindset toolbox.

Summary

- Mind–body therapies are increasingly becoming mainstream and accepted.[24]
- They can give excellent benefits and are as good as medications or interventions for many pain conditions.
- However, most of them do not have the necessary high-quality evidence available to offer them on the NHS/insurers, apart from CBT.
- Have an open mind and explore other mind–body techniques.
- They are generally safe and with very few side effects.
- Consider them to be long-term maintenance options to include in your lifestyle rather than one-off cures or fixes/treatments.

PART 3

Creating a Blueprint for Your Pain

CHAPTER 10

Putting It All Together

WELL DONE FOR making it this far in the book! By now, you hopefully understand that pain is quite a complex sensation and can be determined by multiple factors.

On the positive side, you have by now realised that nociception, when present, can be effectively managed with drugs or interventions. However, there are also treatments that work when there is no nociception, as long as you know that you are now treating a sensitised nervous and immune system.

Having worked through the MINDSET factors in Part 2, let us now see how we can optimise them. You might be thinking that there are just too many choices, but I believe that the more options you are aware of, the better chance you have of taking control of the system and deciding what will help you.

The reality is that:

- The evidence for many interventions, whether drugs, injections or surgery, is low.
- A lot of treatments for chronic pain are not being funded by many insurance bodies and your local NHS.
- Pain is a long-term condition and there are many parts of the pain experience that you can control and play a part in managing.

- In many pain conditions, like low back pain and knee and hip arthritis, the more knowledge you have about your body and health, the better it is, so you know what to add to your plan rather than have no plan at all.

To help you in this process, I have divided the pain strategies you have read about into three main categories:

Done for you (DFY)

This refers to all strategies that generally don't need you to do anything more than follow instructions and be passive. Usually, as in the case of medications and surgery, they are likely to be quite useful if there is clear nociception, such as a swollen knee or fever or infection with blood results that show raised infection markers. However, these treatments generally have side effects that can cause issues. They also tend either to be expensive or have long wait times.

Done with you (DWY)

This refers to those strategies that often involve working with a therapist for a variable period of time, usually 6–12 sessions lasting 30–60 minutes. Some of these therapies involve an element of working on you and then getting you to do some of the exercises, both in the session and at home. These therapies can also be done online, which is convenient. Most of these therapies have fewer side effects when compared to surgery or drugs. However, they are often more time-intensive and can be expensive. The wait times are often long, especially for those therapies that are available on the NHS.

Do it yourself (DIY)

These are the strategies that you do yourself. I think there should be more official resources available to support the DIY approach as sometimes patients don't know exactly what to do, how much to do or how often to do so.

Luckily, since the COVID-19 pandemic, many resources have been made available by both official and non-profit organisations and various technology start-ups. This has been called 'supported self-management'.

Often these techniques are quite safe to do, are reasonably affordable and many times free. They do, however, require a high degree of self-confidence and belief in your health and motivation, and this can sometimes be tough if you are struggling with pain.

Done for you	Done with you	Do it yourself
Medications	Physiotherapy programmes	At-home exercises/ self-massage
Injections and nerve blocks	Pain management programmes	Acupressure dots/ plasters
Surgery of various kinds	Back rehabilitation programmes	TENS machine
Massage/ acupuncture	Functional restoration programmes	Aromatherapy/ equine therapy/ hydrotherapy
Chiropractic manipulation	Breathing techniques/ mindfulness-based stress reduction/most of the therapies mentioned in Chapter 9	Meditation/ mindfulness exercises/breathing techniques

Done for you	Done with you	Do it yourself
Osteopathic therapies	Yoga/tai chi	Yoga/tai chi

You'll see that some of the techniques fall into two categories. Many therapies, like massage or acupuncture, start off as passive exercises but then you may be given some exercises to do at home and a plan may be given for managing other exercises, so it may fit into all three categories.

Now look at the therapies that you have tried. Separate them into those that gave you short-term success and those that didn't work. Similarly for those therapies that you haven't tried, separate them into those techniques you don't want to try at all and those that you might be keen to explore.

Now that you have two groups of techniques – those that gave you short-term success and those that you haven't ever tried but would be willing to explore – answer the questions below:

1. Are they available online?
   Many consultations and physiotherapy and behavioural treatments can now be provided online or via video or telephone.

2. Can they be done only face-to-face/would you prefer it to be face-to-face?
   Treatments like manual therapy, acupuncture or injections are an example.

3. If face-to-face, are they offered as group therapies or individual?

Group therapies are often better as they allow you to take the help of peer support and build a like-minded community of people who understand you and your pain. Individual therapies can be useful for some patients.

4. Are they available locally in your area?
   It must be convenient for you to attend without long commutes and prolonged waiting.

5. What are the ongoing costs?
   The most ideal would be a DWY therapy that empowers/teaches you to gradually do it yourself with support or a direct DIY. As pain is a long-term condition, a pure DWY therapy could be useful, but you need to do it often, which is a cost in the long run.

   Therapies like medications or surgery that are predominantly DFY are most expensive with most side effects. A lot of such treatments are not going to help as well, so even if they are provided by the NHS for free at present, this could always change.

   Finally, fill in the MINDSET template below with your situation as it stands now:

MEDICATIONS: What is your present medication list of pain drugs?	
INTERVENTIONS: Are you waiting for surgery or an injection?	Ask for a chat with your surgeon/pain physician about: B: The benefits of the procedure. Will it give you the outcome you want?

	R: The risks of the procedure. What is the risk of post-surgical pain? A: What are the alternatives to surgery? N: What if we do nothing?
NEUROSCIENCE/STRESS MANAGEMENT: Are you presently under some ongoing personal stress or work-related issues?	
DIET: How much of your daily diet is processed? As a rough guide, anything with more than five ingredients is processed.	Breakfast: Lunch: Dinner: Snacks: Drinks:
SLEEP: How many hours do you sleep right now (weekday and weekend)? What are the reasons for disturbed sleep?	
EXERCISE: Do you get the time/have the ability to do any exercise right now? How many days are you able to do a brisk walk for up to 30 minutes? On average, how many days a week are you doing this?	
THERAPIES: Are you actively doing any mind–body therapies right now? For how long? Are you able to maintain consistency?	

Neuroplasticity

With chronic pain, you will have formed some habits around your response to the pain that you need to untangle and alter in order to form new ones and implement your MINDSET plan. As we saw in Chapter 5, when you develop or change a habit, your brain essentially changes its neural circuits to fire differently. Just by having read this far, your brain has changed and new circuits have formed. This seemingly plastic element of the brain to keep changing throughout life is called neuroplasticity.

If the brain can learn an unnecessary, overprotective pain habit then it can also be unlearned and substituted for a new, safer, more protective habit. This to me is exciting and hopeful!

Every habit has a loop – even your pain. There is often a cue or trigger. When that happens, there is a craving and that prompts a response, which results in a reward. This reward may be a drug that you take to ease the pain. You may not think of it as a reward, but the areas of the brain where opioids and other drugs like alcohol and nicotine act are the same reward systems, so as far as your brain is concerned, by releasing some dopamine as reward it has completed the habit loop.[1]

Habit loop for pain

CUE/TRIGGER $\longrightarrow$ PAIN BEHAVIOUR $\longrightarrow$ AVOIDANCE
CUE/TRIGGER $\longrightarrow$ PAIN MEDICATION $\longrightarrow$ REWARD

Changing the habit means moulding your brain, so it isn't going to be easy but it can be done. Imagine that you wanted to learn a new instrument or language. Unlearning pain is a new language. It will feel hard in the beginning, but, with time, it becomes easier and faster.

Pain is a safety and protection system. Your brain, however, is still in survival mode. An established habit, especially those that seem protective – like not moving when you are in pain – is going to be easier to do. Convincing the brain now to upgrade *and* change needs a slow start, in small steps, with frequent repetition and, most importantly, doing it safely. Remember we talked about nerves that fire together, wire together to form a new neural network (see page 117). Neuroplasticity works on creating these neural networks with your help.

Removing those danger cues and instilling safety cues is particularly important as a first step. This is where doing it in a group or doing it with guidance from a therapist is sometimes useful.

How to form a new habit

The sequence

The American neuroscientist, Andrew Huberman, describes neuroplasticity as a self-directed adaptive plasticity; self-directed because it must be initiated by you. So, when the cue arrives, the brain then must go to the new pathway.[2]

Huberman outlines the steps in the generation of this plasticity. The first step is to focus on the new activity. This can be for a noticeably short time – even one or two minutes – but proper attention and focus needs to be given. This releases a chemical called acetylcholine in the brain.

The increased attention also creates a positive tension in the brain and that releases a chemical called noradrenaline.

This release of the chemicals essentially 'tags' the new nerve circuit. Each time you then do this circuit (repetition), the tags get stronger. When you combine it with sleep these tags are then hardwired, thus making this circuit stronger with time. A final way to seal the deal is to reward this new behaviour, and that can be done with some form of celebration so that it feels satisfying and fun. At a chemical level, this releases dopamine. If this is done in a social setting as a group, it can also release oxytocin and serotonin, all of which improve well-being and hardwire the new circuit and habit.

It takes on average 66 days to form and stabilise a new habit. Consistency, clearly defined goals, tagging the new habit to old ones and having a tracking system and a partner to help you on the journey are some of the ways suggested to form a new habit.[3] You can see how you can now change your pain by using these steps to form a new network.

The motivation myth

Often to do any such repetitive new movements, we think motivation is all that is needed, but, as Stanford professor and author BJ Fogg explains, motivation often comes in waves and is a very fickle and undependable companion.[4] A better option would be to use the following series of steps (adapted from Fogg's method) to match our desires with behaviours we want to do:

Step 1: Clarify a particular outcome/value for your life and a series of goals that map to those values.	For example, reduce my pain to spend more time or go for a walk with family.

Step 2: Explore behaviour options. Brainstorm the various ways to create many ways to achieve a goal.	For example, more time with family could be further subdivided into periods in the morning, afternoon or evening. It can be a school run, mealtime or even an evening walk.
Step 3: Choose a few behaviours that you can potentially easily do. Fogg defines 'Golden Behaviours' as those that you want to do and are easy to do.	For example, sitting at the dinner table and eating with family might be a quick and easy thing to do without flaring your pain while walking may be tricky right now.
Step 4: Start with small steps.	For example, think about just 2–5 minutes of sitting to start with if a whole mealtime is difficult.
Step 5: Find a good prompt.	For example, consider an anchor so that you tie this new habit of sitting for 2–5 minutes with something you already do around that time.
Step 6: Celebrate success.	For example, make sure that you do a high five with your family for having done this. Make sure to reward yourself as this strengthens the habit.

Identify the various behaviours and habits you need to consider changing over time under the following headings and then follow the steps above.

- A new sleep routine.
- A new stress reduction technique.
- A small change in your diet.
- A new exercise/physical activity programme.

Context-dependent

Remember, habits are often context-dependent. This means that you may do something automatically when you are in certain environments. For example, if you have been involved in a road traffic accident, you might feel your muscles tightening up and your breathing getting faster every time you drive or go past that area where the accident occurred. This could apply to certain pain-related postures as well.

If you have back pain, you may be aware of certain postures that you know will trigger that back pain and you take measures to avoid doing that posture. You may have always thought that adopting a certain posture, for example bending or kneeling down, will always bring on muscle spasm and pain. What neuroplasticity tells us is that if your nervous system has learnt a particular circuit then it would already trigger a ready-made pre-prepared plan to tighten the muscle, even before you decide to bend down. It is an overprotective response it has learnt, which can then be unlearnt.

The environment is also important. I often find that this is a problem when patients come to pain management programmes. They learn the habits but are unable to sustain them once they go back home to their old environment, where the triggers are the same and the new habit loop has not had time or the number of repetitions to become strengthened.

James Clear highlights that for any habit to be sustained, it needs to stay very obvious and remain attractive and easy to do while satisfying. Once you have formed a new habit, make sure that you:

- Join a group (online/social media) to support you and keep you going.
- Invest in a tracker system or technology app to keep measuring and reinforcing.
- Keep rewarding yourself with mini celebrations to keep it fun and enjoyable.
- Don't worry if you 'fall off the wagon'. It happens as the brain is learning.
- Consider making it part of a ritual so it becomes almost natural, like brushing your teeth on waking up.

Are you patient and compassionate with yourself as you rewire your plastic brain? It takes between 44 and 66 repetitions for learning to become wired.[5]

Creating a Flare-up Plan

A flare-up is very common and can be a combination of increased pain and reduced activity, accompanied by mood changes. It is not to be feared and, indeed, it gives you the opportunity to practise the skills that you have learnt. It is the equivalent of doing the driving test after having learnt the theory and taken the lessons. You will make mistakes, which is fine.

I would suggest that you keep a pain log or tracker on your smartphone to identify some links between possible triggers and flare-ups. Keep track of how it resolved and what you did to resolve it. This way, you get to be your own Sherlock

Holmes in knowing what works for you and what can make it worse. This also allows you to plan.

Flare-up checklist

Questions to consider when you experience a pain flare-up:

1. Have you been involved in an injury or surgery? Yes/No
2. Is there a visible swelling in any part of the body with increased temperature or fever or other signs of infection? Yes/No
3. Have you been overdoing something? Yes/No
4. Is there a source of stress; emotional or physical, thoughts or people? Yes/No
5. Has there been a change to your diet in the preceding few days? Yes/No

If the answers to questions 1 and 2 are no, then your pain is unlikely to be due to nociception, so medications and interventions are likely to be unsuccessful. In such situations, reaching out to your MINDSET toolkit to practise the techniques that soothe and calm the oversensitised nervous system is the main aim.

How you manage these flare-ups will also determine what you do with each future flare-up, how long it lasts and its severity as the brain keeps learning each time. Manage it well and you will find that future flare-ups are easier to deal with, last a shorter time and are not so severe.

While doing this, you might have found activities or exercises that are more personal for you, so the techniques will change from person to person. However, a few common techniques that I would suggest are:

- **A breathing technique:** Noted author and GP Dr Rangan Chatterjee suggests five simple breathing techniques, one of which is the 3–4–5 technique.[6] It is simple and effective and helps move you from the threat to soothe state. You breathe in for three seconds, hold your breath for four seconds and breathe out slowly for five seconds. Doing this for three minutes significantly reduces stress and consequently pain during a flare-up. An alternative would be box breathing.
- **Do a body scan** (see page 248).
- **Reassess your plans** for the rest of the day.

Flare-up strategy	Planned techniques
Relaxation	<ul><li>3–4–5 breathing technique</li><li>Body scan</li><li>Progressive muscular relaxation</li><li>Medications if above don't work</li></ul>
Distraction	<ul><li>Music</li><li>Movies</li><li>Social connection</li><li>Games on phone/virtual reality app</li></ul>
Activity level	<ul><li>Note activity pattern that works</li><li>Reduce activity but don't completely stop</li><li>Minimal stretches and short walks</li><li>Pacing techniques</li></ul>

Mood management	<ul><li>Positive affirmations</li><li>Meditation</li><li>Visualisation and imagery</li><li>Talking to friends/seeking connection</li></ul>

THE 80:20 RULE

Wayne Jonas prefers to call the placebo response (which I introduced to you on page 76) the meaning response. In a compelling fashion, he shows that any of the treatments you get in traditional biomedical care account for only 20 per cent of the healing you need. The remaining 80 per cent comes from the highly personal interpretation of the meaning response that is unique to you. True integrative health means you need to take charge of some of your long-term health issues and work with your specialist to find a safe, effective and affordable way forward. It should fit with your 80 per cent and not the 20 per cent you will get from the hospital specialists. The pain-free mindset forms part of the plan for you to embrace the 80 per cent that will do most of the healing for you.

With any pain that you experience, always remember that there might be some nociceptive elements that *may* respond to a drug or surgery/injection, but always factor in the experience of 'pain' and the emotional involvement to give you a wider set of techniques.

This book hopefully has given you the set of tools to manage and understand all the other facets of pain that are not going to be helped by more injections, surgery or medications.

The new strategies you learnt in this chapter:

- take advantage of the principle that the nervous and immune systems constantly can learn and change and adapt
- encourage you to be more curious and less fearful about your pain
- show you newer and safer techniques to try to become pain-free

However, I also believe that this is not something that should just be left to you alone. It is important that you get access to many of the treatments that I have outlined in other chapters. Obviously, some of these will not have the level of evidence right now that is required for the NHS to provide or for insurers to authorise, but this is something that we as healthcare professionals are actively researching and getting the evidence so that patients like you benefit.

If you feel that this book has given you the knowledge and confidence and you want to upgrade and learn new skills, then a pain management programme will be for you, and this is the focus of the next chapter.

Summary

- There is patchy and poor availability of many pain relief techniques on the NHS, so it is important for you to make a list of what can work for you.
- The aim for you should be to learn a technique so that you can feel confident to make it part of your pain-free mindset backpack.

- The systems and habits you learn are going to decide how you overcome pain successfully rather than just idealistic goals.
- Neuroplasticity means that the nervous system can unlearn pain just as it learnt to amplify pain.
- Like any skill, frequent repetition helps you become much better.
- Flare-ups/relapses can happen in the process of rewiring, so a flare-up plan is essential.

CHAPTER 11

Pain Management/
Rehabilitation Programmes

MOST PAIN CLINICS in the UK and internationally talk about pain management programmes (PMPs), also called rehabilitation programmes, functional restoration programmes or well-being programmes depending on which part of the world you live in. You may have done one yourself and it could have been a life-changer, or you may not have found it useful for you. These are often provided as the last treatment once all other strategies, including multiple surgeries (sometimes), have been done.

In my opinion, I think we have got it completely wrong and it should be the other way around. What gets taught in a PMP often should be the first set of strategies that are explained to you and you should be aware of.

A PMP is a **skills- and habit-building** framework. It is a planned intervention lasting for six to eight weeks that aims to train the mind and start the process of rewiring your nervous system through a variety of behavioural and movement techniques. Most of them are run by psychologists and physiotherapists/occupational therapists/nurses and doctors, and should be available in your local NHS hospital.

The core framework may be CBT- or ACT-based (see pages 243 and 244), and they include mindfulness- and compassion-based exercises. Cognitive and behavioural skills are important as pain is often accompanied by mood changes in most patients.[1] Goal-setting based on your values and what you want is an important part of the programme. Pacing is also an important skill that you learn as we know that exposure to a new movement or technique can be difficult. PMPs also provide education and advice around sleep hygiene, physical activity regimes, diet and other lifestyle advice, as appropriate.

Whether you do them online or face-to-face, all healthcare professionals delivering the PMP first establish rapport with you and the other group members, before getting you to understand the following three important skills:[2]

1. Control breathing

The initial focus in most NHS programmes is often the body and to learn about the body via a body scan and breathing techniques.

Breathing is one of the few automatic or semi-automatic processes that we can have some control over. We can't control our digestion, we can't control our heart rate to a certain extent, we can't control the hormone release, but breathing is something that we can control.

When we combine the body and the breath, we can stabilise or bring the mind to an equilibrium. Once the mind is stabilised, we move on to the thoughts and behaviours. If you learn the skill to do this, then it will give you the ability to change breathing and not get influenced when negative thoughts or sounds happen.

2. Modify and change the old response to pain

When you understand how your body responds, you then develop the ability to know how to modify your old response and change to a more powerful and safer new response.

PMPs raise awareness of the automatic thoughts, patterns or tendencies and make those subconscious or unconscious automatic thoughts come into the conscious realm. Once you become aware, you then have a choice on how to respond to them.

Do you want to do it the old way or do you want to try to do it in an open, non-judgemental way?

3. Make new habits and embrace neuroplasticity

If you want to do things a new way, you need to be willing to be open and curious. A growth mindset is needed, which means that mistakes are to be considered as part of learning rather than worrying about them. Similarly, doing a new thing might in the short term feel like the pain has worsened. However, sticking with it is important.

Most programmes also provide homework because the aim is to empower you to move into DIY. **Remember, the programme is getting you on the first rung of the self-management ladder with support and will give you a set of skills. It is up to you to reinforce the good habit to make it the default behaviour.**

ADVANTAGES OF PMPS

1. They are often done in groups. The evidence around skill and habit formation shows that doing this in a group is useful on many levels (see page 231). Meeting

---

other people with similar issues means that you can gain support and find accountability partners.

2. We know that dealing with pain alone is a major problem. The group setting of PMPs reduces the isolation and frustration that can cause helplessness and loss of self-esteem.

3. Learning from others. Often having peer support and knowing how someone else similar to you has done a particular activity can make you more confident in trying it than healthcare professionals simply advising it. The 'lived experience' you have is an expertise that you can share with others to help change their pain journey.

4. Practitioners try to make the experience of gaining new skills with your mind an enjoyable one rather than a hard task.

5. Often an educational component is there along with the movement, which helps clarify the choices available to you.

6. From an economic perspective, as long as all the components are there, doing a PMP could be more cost-effective as it will give you all the tools in one programme, rather than you attending multiple different therapies.

Outline of a Typical Programme

In my hospital, our ten-week PMP is called 'XPLORE', and it has both CBT and ACT principles. After patients have answered some baseline questionnaires, they follow the framework below:

Sessions 1 and 2	Introduction and education around pain science and the changes to the anatomy and physiology in chronic pain. Introduction to breathing techniques and the concept of the threat/drive and soothe systems in all of us.
Sessions 3, 4, 5 and 6	Further work around mindfulness and being flexible psychologically. Patients are encouraged to be open, and aware of their thoughts, pain, feelings and actions. Links are made between the values they want and the actions they need to take. Acceptance of some of the sensations is also taught while recognising some unhelpful thoughts. Use of mental imagery and visualisation and ongoing movement and physical activity is encouraged.
Sessions 7 and 8	Compassion is introduced and various activities and exercises are taught to enhance the mindfulness movement and exposure to fear-based avoidance.
Sessions 9 and 10	Helpful and unhelpful communication styles are looked at and taught. A flare-up plan is created and populated, which can then be used by the group members for future reference (see page 278).

HOW TO ACCESS PMPS

In the first instance you should contact your GP so that they can refer you to the local pain service that runs such a programme. While I have outlined the benefits of doing it in a group, and indeed more than 90 per cent of such programmes are group-based, there are still options to get it individually, especially if you are not comfortable in group settings or you live far away and cannot make it regularly due to personal circumstances.

Both options can be available privately and there are also smartphone apps and other programmes that are quite affordable and still accessible. Many programmes, whether they are face-to-face or online, will provide you with other resources, in terms of videos, audios and written work. Since the COVID-19 pandemic, there has been a huge rise in online PMPs that can cater to individual needs as well.

Are You Ready for a PMP?

This is often a difficult question to answer, both for the patient and the therapist who is assessing you. Many of the face-to-face programmes that are run as groups have long wait times and have been poorly funded so there are not enough of them around. They are also intensive and do need you to commit to their time frames and weekly sessions.

Aiming to harness your neuroplasticity is a lifelong skill and the advantages in doing so are tremendous. Nevertheless, many people find that they are not ready and end up dropping out after the first few sessions, or sometimes after the first, when they realise that this isn't a cure.

Those who are motivated can be more ready for an online PMP or even doing some of the DIY approaches I have outlined in the Resources section (see page 313). Those who are less motivated may need more support and advice first to understand their pain before a PMP.

American psychology professors James Prochaska and Carlo DiClemente suggest that most people go through a set of six stages in their mind when taking on a new behaviour or habit.[3] With regards to your chronic pain, I have outlined what that means below. Which stage are you in?

Stage 1: Pre-contemplation You think that there must be a cure and quick fix for the pain, that one more intervention or new drug will take away the pain forever. You often feel like there is no ability to control the pain. You know what's causing the pain.	You are likely to be still in the DFY category. You are not *yet* ready to change/manage and are not open to new ideas. You will need specialist help and more support in clarifying your beliefs. **You are not yet ready for a PMP.** **Action needed from your healthcare professional (HCP): More awareness and education for you.**
Stage 2: Contemplation You are more open and curious. You are willing to weigh up the risk and benefits. You are starting to doubt some of those theories you had.	You are ready for a DWY approach. You will need more active support in self-managing and improving confidence in your own skills. **You are likely to be ready for a PMP and the pain-free mindset journey.** **Action needed from your HCP: Helping with change.**

Stage 3: Preparation You are ready to engage. You need to undertake more reading and looking up new knowledge and understanding about pain, mood and health.	You are ready for DWY and supported DIY. You will benefit from the right support and signposting. You have some knowledge and skills, but will benefit from support. You are ready to accept new ideas. **You are ready for a PMP.** **Action needed from your HCP:** Right signposting.
Stage 4: Action You are doing the work and learning the skills. You are able to do new and multiple behaviours and have a full understanding of your own role in pain control.	You are ready for **DIY**. You will benefit from more timely support and provision of the right resources, knowledge, confidence and skills. **You could benefit from a top-up of a PMP or online options.** **Action needed from your HCP:** Signpost to online resources.
Stage 5: Maintenance You are learning new and better skills, trying new techniques of self-management of pain and new habits are now embedded. Neuroplasticity is complete.	You know when you need help (DWY) and when to employ DIY. **You can access resources as needed and are fully engaged with your own health and medications.** **Action needed from your HCP:** Signpost to online resources. You can help other patients.

Stage 6: Relapse	
Flare-ups can occur in pain. You sometimes fall back to old behaviours of seeking medications/ interventions.	This can often happen in pain control. You will generally improve and get better after any flare-up. However, you will need support and reviewing/refining of the plan. You will benefit from some DWY and encouragement and support to move through Steps 2–5. **You may benefit from a top-up of a PMP where provided.**

Action needed from HCP: Reassure and avoid overtreatment and support renewal of self-care. Flare-up plan revision and enhancement. |

Summary

- PMPs are fundamentally an opportunity for you to build new skills and feel confident in overcoming your pain.
- Control of your breathing, modifying the old response and learning new patterns are core skills you will learn from a PMP.
- PMPs are approved and available on the NHS. They are available both online and face-to-face.
- Identifying which stage of change you are in will help you decide whether you are ready for a PMP.
- It is a time commitment, but is well worth it for the lifetime of change it will bring.

CHAPTER 12

The Future

AT LEAST ONCE a week, I see an article in the newspaper or online about a new magic wand and hope for chronic pain. Most of this is hype and generally serves as clickbait for that webpage or magazine. However, amidst the noise, there are some interesting and potentially fantastic treatments that are being actively researched. Some of these are already available for trial in the UK while many are still in various phases of being tested.

The good thing is that, while some of the treatments are aimed at those patients where nociception is a bigger player, most of them are looking to calm the nervous and immune systems that amplify pain.

Medicinal cannabis

While cannabis has been around for thousands of years, the last 70–80 years have seen it being viewed as a dangerous gateway drug with huge problems. While all that may still be the case, there is also no doubt that it does work for a wide variety of medical conditions and especially many forms of neuropathic and nociplastic pain. What we now understand is that, alongside our sympathetic (fight/flight) and parasympathetic (rest/digest) nervous systems, we have also got our own endocannabinoid system (balance/harmony) and we produce our own internal cannabis.[1]

The cannabis receptor (CB1) is the most common receptor in the body and it is thought that the endocannabinoid system is responsible for the overall balance and homeostasis of the human body. The fact that our brain/body immune system (glial cells) has cannabis receptors (CB2) may also point to why cannabis seems to work for certain kinds of nociplastic pain. While, at the time of writing, the evidence for its use is still not considered high-quality, I have no doubt that this will change over the next few years.

Glial modulators (microglia and astrocytes)

Since we understood that pain can be amplified within the spinal cord and the brain, we have realised that our immune cells (activated microglia) are a key factor in chronic pain and newer drugs and therapies to inhibit or reduce the activation are being trialled. Promising candidates already available are an antibiotic called minocycline and medicinal cannabis. Other drugs being actively studied include diabetic drugs like metformin and rosiglitazone.[2] Non-drug options, like omega-3 PUFA, turmeric, bacopa (an Ayurvedic herb) and many Asian spices, all reduce the inflammatory chemicals that are released from activated glia.[3] Even fasting and ketogenic diets can modulate the microglia alongside techniques such as yoga and meditation.

Immune therapies

Many inflammatory chemicals (cytokines) are often released into arthritic joints and also within the nervous system by the immune cells in some cases of chronic pain. This has meant trials of monoclonal antibodies, just as is the case for rheumatoid arthritis. A few intravenous drugs are being trialled for some kinds of arthritic pain.

Regenerative therapies

These are a broad category of injection-based interventions that are becoming quite popular. Older forms like prolotherapy have been popular for several decades in pain conditions where the problem is suspected to be laxity of the ligaments or soft tissues around the joints. Injections with such agents would provoke the body's immune system to complete the healing job, thus reducing pain. The newer form of regenerative therapy includes taking some of your blood and separating the growth factors and blood cells and injecting the platelet-rich plasma (PRP) into the painful area.[4] Since the platelets contain growth factors, healing is promoted and pain can be reduced. Of course, this is most useful when nociception is still the main reason for the pain.

Mesenchymal stem cells

These are cells that are found in your bone marrow that retain the ability to differentiate and make and repair various tissues in the body. You can think of them as your potential transformer cells that often can release chemicals that promote repair and calm the immune and nervous systems. Several animal and human studies are ongoing to see its benefit in a variety of chronic autoimmune disease conditions as well as back and neuropathic pain.[5]

Transcranial magnetic stimulation (TMS)

This is a non-invasive safe technique that is being used for nociplastic pain. It involves the creation of a magnetic field that is then applied across the patient's head and it passes through to the superficial regions of the brain and changes the way the connections fire.[6] It also reduces the activation of the microglia and astrocytes. It has been used for a wide number of pain conditions. The evidence is still not adequate to know who it will definitely work on.

Neuromodulation

This is a broad umbrella term for any kind of electrical therapy technique that involves placing a thin wire into the spinal cord or brain to provide small pulses of electricity into various parts of the nervous system. This is already available on the NHS for certain kinds of neuropathic pain and the evidence base is increasing for other kinds of nociceptive pain. It may be dampening the signals going to the brain and it may also be changing the functioning of the glia in the spinal cord and reducing inflammation at that level. Apart from stimulating the spinal cord and brain, the vagus nerve also responds to a variety of stimulation techniques. Vagal nerve stimulators are being tried for a variety of pain and mood disorders and the principle again is influencing the immune system of the brain and modifying the neuroinflammation.

Virtual reality (VR)

Increasingly more affordable, VR has now been used for many acute pain conditions and is being trialled for several chronic pain problems. VR works by primarily distraction techniques but it is being used to focus our attention away from the pain (focus shifting) and also building skills (teaching breathing techniques through reminders or learning about pain in an immersive, interactive manner).[7] More work needs to be done in identifying the right kind of patient and content; however, the opportunities are exciting and the risk of side effects at this time are low.

Epigenetics

Epigenetics literally means 'on top' of our genes. Simply put, we realise that genes and their hereditary nature are not our entire story. If DNA in our cells gives the instructions for what to produce, epigenetics refers to those factors that can literally switch 'on and off' the genes so that it can change what finally gets produced by the body. These epigenetic factors can come from the environment, the stress we face, the food we eat or the chemicals we get exposed to. So, while genetics may load our health 'gun', epigenetics is what pulls the trigger. This has implications for our life and chronic pain because, by modifying our lifestyle and diet/nutrition, physical activity and stress, we can change our script![8]

Digital trackers/wearables

These have almost become mainstream. The technology, however, is still evolving and right now there is more chance for error. As the data that feeds into the software becomes significant, accuracy will improve. More importantly, these digital devices can become your accountability coach and habit tracker, which is genuinely exciting as it means you can bring about behaviour change in a way you want to when you want to. Apps for anxiety and mood management have become immensely popular and habit apps are also being adopted to aid this process.

WHAT YOU CAN DO

- **Get empowered.** If you want to reduce your pain and get back to health, it's important that you focus not just on the treatments that are done for you passively, but also use this book and the tools you have learnt so that you feel more empowered, have confidence and take control in managing your pain and overcoming it.
- **Educate others.** A big reason for the epidemic of poor pain management is the lack of awareness and training amongst medical providers around the various techniques that can be used for pain management. Pain is complex *but* that is no excuse for providing poor-quality care or wrong information or continuing to believe in flawed, outdated science. You can use this book to discuss your pain plan more knowledgeably with your healthcare professional or, better still, gift it to them!
- **Support appropriate funding.** We tend to pay thousands of pounds for a surgery because we think it's a fix-it. However, an average of one in five does not work. There should be a mechanism to fund the broad integrative techniques as suggested in this book through your local pain service. You can bring this to the attention of your local MP or Clinical Commissioning Group (CCG)/Primary Care Network (PCN). A longer-term rehabilitation plan with more realistic outcomes based upon function and quality of life needs to be supported.

Benefits for Society

Understanding the principles of the pain-free mindset and practising it can be beneficial, not just for you but also for society and healthcare in general.

Promoting salutogenesis

Introduced by professor of medical sociology, Aaron Antonovsky, salutogenesis looks at the factors needed to support human health and well-being, rather than our present biomedical model of 'curing' disease.[9] While there are understandable privacy concerns, our phones have the potential to enable this. They can be a central hub that integrates the overall aspects of health data from you, such as body weight, food intake and mode of physical activity. This information can be available to your specialist, who can then create personalised plans incorporating all aspects of the pain-free mindset. Behaviour change can be facilitated and, if we can help with small, quantifiable, visible and measurable changes like this over a period of time, I am sure that will be responsible for a major transformation of healthcare.

Newer understanding of the power of the brain

The knowledge of neuroplasticity and the adaptive capacity of the brain and spinal cord and the adoption of the growth mindset inherent in the pain-free mindset approach needs dissemination throughout various educational institutions at multiple levels (schools, universities and medical schools in particular), along with other healthcare professional education settings, such as chiropractic, nursing or physiotherapy schools.

The present model of thinking about pain is wrong. It is also responsible for some of the worst and unnecessary healthcare spending that we have seen in the last three decades. If this is to change in any meaningful way, then there is an urgent need for the educational sector, especially healthcare education, to address this deficit appropriately and quickly.

While it is heartening to note that universities and schools are increasing exposure of young people to various lifestyle and well-being strategies, the beneficial effects of the right education about pain, the growth mindset and neuroplasticity at this age can last a lifetime.

Organisational support

At an organisational level, it is vital to recognise the link between mind and body and appreciate the importance and difference between nociception and pain. At present, insurers support short-term nociceptive interventions such as surgery/injections, but do not recognise or support mind–body therapies for pain on a longer-term basis like they do for cancer treatment. Both are long-term conditions with a significant impact on quality of life.

The NHS should also be encouraging habit and behaviour change. The ability to incentivise and use the reward mechanisms to change habits is a good strategy to encourage employees to be more mindful and to take more active control of their health and well-being.

Community and grassroots campaigns

At the local government and public policy level, we need to improve education around pain science. This has been achieved quite remarkably in Australian public health campaigns along with researcher initiatives like Professor Lorimer Moseley's Pain Revolutions. Locally in the UK, Flipping Pain is a joint initiative between Connect Health and the NHS Teesside University to explore a similar grassroots educational campaign to residents of Lincolnshire.

Similar such initiatives need to occur on a more national scale. We know that often evidence from research can take 10–15 years for the benefits to be translated to patients. This was in the era when social media and Internet use wasn't widespread. Seeing how knowledge about newer drugs and treatments/therapies and vaccines were fast-tracked during the COVID-19 pandemic, this kind of delay in years is no longer acceptable.

Access for all

The relative lack of evidence for some of the mind–body therapies and nutritional strategies and sleep/exercise techniques should be the subject of honest discussion and debate between patients and their caregivers and tailored to the needs of the local population. Data and the relative prevalence of some conditions versus others can be obtained locally and we could work with other voluntary groups and charities to make some of these treatments more accessible to patients. After all, patients who suffer from post-cancer-related chemotherapy-induced pain can often get access to mind–body therapies like aromatherapy and acupuncture, which help both their mood and their pain. Why should this not be offered to patients struggling and suffering from non-cancer-related pain?

The Challenge and the Solution

I understand that transforming or changing the outlook of an entire society will not be easy nor will it be achieved overnight. Yet this is possible, and it is being attempted in many parts of the world.

Value-based healthcare

Providing patients with best value in terms of quality of care, efficiency and effectiveness, both in terms of cost as well as patient satisfaction, is a definition of value-based healthcare. American integrative physician and pain doctor, Wayne Jonas, has been able to incorporate the principles of mind–body medicine and various treatments into his local healthcare system.[10] He collects a detailed assessment of the patient's 'healing' environment that helps his team understand what is relevant to the psychosocial aspects of that patient.

Community engagement

While the Internet can seem to shorten distances, a person in pain still lives, works and interacts with their local community. Empowering the patient to seek help from their community and working with the local community/council to provide resources like social prescribing can integrate a patient with the community and strengthen social bonds.

In his book *The Community Cure*, health economist and activist James Maskell focuses on the problems of loneliness, non-communicable diseases and the lack of a more progressive, participatory and personalised medicine approach.[11] Improving connections and forming local peer support networks is a worthwhile suggestion to consider.

Trauma-informed and responsive care

For successful implementation of value-based sustainable healthcare, the adoption of trauma-informed care is essential.[12] When you face big and small traumatic events in your life (major surgery/cancer/abuse/bullying, etc.), the individual way in which you experience those (and your past experiences) will shape how adverse the effects are going to be for you. When these traumas are coupled with environmental factors (poor nutrition and low social connection/support/resilience), they can cause stress and neuroinflammation and worsen any pain. Realising and recognising this and responding to it appropriately is vital. Being sensitive to this and working to create a personalised responsive plan that addresses all aspects carefully and compassionately is the true way to achieve a pain-free mindset.

COVID-19 and Pain

We know that the COVID-19 pandemic has had a tremendous impact on our lives. As a traumatic event, this is a major trauma for most people with impacts not only on physical but also on mental health. There have been social consequences of this (isolation of lockdown, recession, redundancy and unemployment, and increased abuse/violence), all of which are going to be potential stressors and sensitise the nervous and immune systems.

The virus itself causes widespread immune overactivity and can damage many organs. While most people do recover, we are now realising that a sizeable proportion (one in ten) are likely to be left with their immune and nervous systems oversensitised. This can happen in anyone, but those with previous medical issues, those who have needed ICU or had organ system damage acutely are more at risk.[13] 'LongCOVID' or 'post-COVID syndrome' is the condition where people continue to suffer from debilitating fatigue, pain and brain fog/worsened mental health and various other symptoms 12 weeks after their acute infection. It is still being actively researched whether this is a feature of ongoing neuroinflammation, residual virus or organ damage by the 'cytokine storm'.

Clinics have now been established to assess and investigate such patients, irrespective of whether they needed hospitalisation or not. A small percentage of LongCOVID sufferers will have some evidence of damage to their heart muscle or lung tissue. However, for everyone suffering with LongCOVID, their most common symptoms of fatigue, pain, increased anxiety and breathing issues are going to be due to an overactivated neuroimmune system. If there is added contribution from adverse traumatic events like isolation and unemployment, unhealthy fast foods or decreased physical activity with disturbed sleep, then the chances of pain amplification are a lot higher due to further sensitisation of the system and all the factors I have mentioned in previous chapters.

As you have learnt throughout this book, the management and long-term sure-fire way of calming the sensitised system is to pay attention to the pillars of lifestyle: nutrition, physical activity, sleep, relaxation (mind–body) techniques, social connection and community. While a vaccination programme is underway, we know that vaccines are not a cure for COVID-19 and LongCOVID doesn't have a proven drug-based cure as yet. Therefore, paying attention to and including all the essential components of the pain-free mindset in managing your pain and fatigue is more important than ever.

A lot of the techniques and advice that I have discussed throughout this book are being delivered through the long COVID clinics, with modules on sleep, pacing and nutrition, alongside activity/breathing and relaxation techniques. Using the techniques taught in these clinics alongside the pain-free mindset toolbox will ensure that you can recover quicker.

Summary

- There are a number of newer treatment strategies that have the potential to vastly improve pain.
- The community can be a potential source of support for helping with pain.
- A trauma-informed care approach is essential for personalised and sustainable healthcare in the future
- LongCOVID can be improved by using many of the pain-free mindset strategies.

Conclusion

IT WAS A dark, dreary New Year's Eve and Pete had turned 31. The year was 1994. The back pain that had now plagued him for three years had made his life a living hell and it wouldn't change. He found himself contemplating ending it all. He thought to himself, 'What is the point of it all? There must be something more to life than all of this.'

A painter and interior decorator by profession, Pete's backache had started after a routine twisting movement while at work. He could not recollect any trigger or trauma, but it left him struggling to manage it.

Like most of us in the nineties, when medical knowledge was expanding but probably not adequately and certainly not in the right direction, Pete sought help from his GP and then a specialist on how to fix his pain. In his own words he 'continued doctor shopping and physio shopping and health professional shopping of any kind; anyone who could promise me a fix for my back pain. Each massage and acupuncture session that I had, I went in with the assumption that this was going to be the treatment that was going to get rid of my pain forever.'

Each session left him feeling hopeless. He had steroid injections that didn't work. The pain had started to affect his mood and self-esteem, depression set in along with sleep disturbance, and he was not able to work.

Eventually he got referred to the pain management programme in his local NHS hospital. In those times it was one of a kind and there were very few such programmes around the country. According to Pete, the pain management programme changed his life. It made him understand what he could do to look after his pain, and for the first time he got the confidence and the introduction to the skills that he needed to look after himself and gain control of his pain.

It was while he was doing this programme that he understood the difference between nociception and pain. He realised that all the professionals he was going to see at that time were conflating both and were hoping that if they treated the nociception then the pain would go away. Understanding that he could separate them and focus on activities that he could do and functions of life that he could still enjoy gave him the power to work on the pain and realise that nociception wasn't the issue.

It's now coming up to 27 years since that year and in these last two decades Pete Moore has become an advocate and the poster child for self-management. He has realised that pain can be overcome and it does not depend on medications and interventions. In fact, he is not taking any medications. He went back to work in 2000. During his period of being off sick and on benefits, he reckons that it cost the state a little over £350,000 to look after him and pay for the treatments he got.

His back pain hasn't fully gone away and the passage of time has brought on issues like arthritis and prostate cancer, all of which he has bravely managed. But the implementation of self-management has meant that he has never relied on medications or healthcare professionals to 'get rid' of his pain. Breaking away from that fundamental flawed premise of seeking a passive approach of medication or a surgical quick fix gave Pete an opportunity to view his pain in a different way. He realised that he had a number of options that he could use to bring down the pain and, in some cases, eliminate it completely in order to go back to some of the activities he loved.

He can now go bike riding and for long drives, and you can check him out on his social media profile. He's a lifelong Gunners fan and continues to follow them avidly. Most importantly, in the last two decades, his work on self-management and the creation of the 'Pain Toolkit' has seen multiple translations and adaptations of his work in more than one hundred countries around the world. His collaborations with fellow patient advocates as well as other healthcare professionals have ushered in a new much-needed era of support for the patient in chronic pain.

Pete Moore's story of overcoming his pain by embodying the principles of self-management is something that we all can aspire to. You, as the reader of this book and having come this far, now are in the same position that Pete was when he finished the pain management programme, but you have much better access to the most state-of-the-art knowledge on pain.

Various options are available to you to trial and create a plan that will work for you. Often the problem has been an ability to find good, high-quality, trustworthy people, websites or organisations to go to for help. This is often a major stumbling block for members of the public because they do not know whether the information that they are reading on the Internet is reliable or trustworthy. Hopefully this book will give you confidence by giving you the knowledge.

The main issue is whether you are ready to believe and realise that you have the power to change and overcome your pain. If you can accept that, we are in a much better place to help create more Pete Moores than ever before. The power of neuroplasticity and the ability of the brain to rewire itself can happen. If you can do it in the right way and be aided by good support and lifestyle measures that can reverse the effect that stress and inflammation can have on the nervous and immune systems, then there is a very good chance that you can overcome your pain.

If chronic pain has been a part of your life up to now and this book has helped you understand your options and choices, then that means it has given you control. If you have control, you can work with your pain and get your way. Once you see that pain is a problem that you have, not someone else's problem to fix, then you become the decision-making authority. You get to choose what you want to do.

If you are open to learning the skills of self-management and knowing more about your treatment options, then you will be able to decide how much you can control on your own and when you need to seek help from healthcare professionals. This is what this book has set out to do – to give you the knowledge and the confidence that you can overcome your pain and have a much better quality of life and reduce the suffering when you adopt the pain-free mindset.

Resources

Further reading

The following books may be of interest to you:

- Paul Christo, *Aches and Gains* (Bull Publishing, 2017)
- Shelly Prosko and Marlysa Sullivan, *Yoga and Science in Pain Care* (Singing Dragon, 2019)
- Joe Tatta, *Heal Your Pain Now* (Da Capo Lifelong Books, 2017)
- Sean Young, *Stick With It* (Penguin Life, 2018)

If you want to read and understand more about mind–body techniques then please check out the following books, as well as the resource by ATrain Education:

- Margaret Caudill-Slosberg, *Managing Pain Before It Manages You* (Guilford Press, 2016)
- Frances Cole, Helen Macdonald, Catherine Carus and Hazel Howden-Leach, *Overcoming Chronic Pain* (Robinson Press, 2020)
- Cindy Perlin, *The Truth About Chronic Pain Treatments* (Morning Light Books, 2015)

- Atrain Education, 'Complementary, Alternative, and Integrative Therapies', available at: atrainceu.com/content/16-complementary-alternative-and-integrative-therapies

Online resources

Mindfulness apps

- Aura: aurahealth.io
- Breethe: breethe.com
- Buddhify: buddhify.com
- Calm: calm.com
- Headspace: headspace.com
- Palouse mindfulness-based stress reduction: palouse mindfulness.com
- Sattva: sattva.life
- Smiling Mind: smilingmind.com.au

Diet and nutrition

- Gluten-free foods: healthline.com/nutrition/gluten-food-list#foods-to-eat
- Glycaemic index: glycemicindex.com
- That Sugar Movement: thatsugarmovement.com
- The dirty dozen: pan-uk.org/dirty-dozen-and-clean-fifteen

Sleep

- NHS sleep self-assessment: assets.nhs.uk/tools/self-assessments/index.mob.html?variant=72
- Sleep Cycle: sleepcycle.com
- Sleepio: sleepio.com

- Sleepscore: sleepscore.com
- The Sleep Council 30-day sleep plan: sleepcouncil.org. uk/advice-support/sleep-tools/30-day-sleep-plan
- The Sleep Foundation good sleep hygiene: sleepfoundation.org/articles/sleep-hygiene

Mind–body therapies

- Body scan: soundcloud.com/diarmuiddenneny/body-scan/s-xsDyB (with permission from Diarmuid Denneny, physiotherapy lead, Pain Management Centre, UCLH)
- NHS guide to yoga: nhs.uk/live-well/exercise/guide-to-yoga
- Physiotherapy Pain Association: ppa.csp.org.uk
- The Mindful Word mindfulness-based stress reduction exercises: themindfulword.org/2012/mbsr-mindfulness-based-stress-reduction

Further online support

- Aches and Gains: podcasts.apple.com/ie/podcast/aches-and-gains-with-dr-paul-christo/id1233732954 American pain physician Paul Christo interviews various celebrities about chronic pain and how they have overcome their pain.
- Empowered Beyond Pain: ebppodcast.podomatic.com A great podcast channel by Peter O'Sullivan's group talking all things pain-related.
- How does your brain respond to pain?: youtube.com/watch?v=I7wfDenj6CQ A quick animated five-minute video from Karen Davis on the experience of pain.

- Integrative Pain Science Institute: integrative painscienceinstitute.com/podcasts
  An excellent resource for patients with regard to nutrition for chronic pain and podcasts around integrative pain management by Joe Tatta.
- Pain-Ed: pain-ed.com/public/patient-stories-2
  An excellent website with numerous patient stories of recovery from chronic pain.
- Retrain Pain Foundation: retrainpain.org
  A collection of one-minute videos on pain and its complexity.
- Why things hurt: youtube.com/watch?v=gwd-wLdIHjs &t=27s
  A very entertaining TED Talk by Lorimer Moseley about the neurobiology of pain.

Pain management programmes

Inpatient

There are a few NHS and private centres that offer inpatient/high-intensity/online group programmes that can often be for three to four weeks, such as:

- Bath Centre for Pain Services: bathcentreforpainservices. nhs.uk/what-we-do/how-to-refer
- Guy's and St Thomas': guysandstthomas.nhs.uk/our-services/pain/input/patients/programmes.aspx
- Optimise, Oxford University Hospitals: ouh.nhs.uk/ optimise

- Royal National Orthopaedic Hospital: rnoh.nhs.uk/services/rehabilitation-and-therapy/pain-self-management-patients
- Real Health: realhealth.uk
- Vitality360: vitality360.co.uk

Online

- Curable: curablehealth.com (DIY)
  The latest and one of the more scientifically advanced platforms, this American start-up embraces mind–body medicine, and offers online group support for as long as 12 weeks.
- Flippin' Pain®: flippinpain.co.uk (DIY)
  This is a public health campaign that is keen to raise awareness by grassroots pain education and by showing the most recent pain research in a friendly animated form.
- My Live Well With Pain: my.livewellwithpain.co.uk (DIY)
  Another excellent resource, this website offers the ten footsteps approach for patients and healthcare professionals, and has collated several educational resources for free.
- MyPain®: mypain.uk (DWY to DIY)
  This is the latest and most advanced UK-based technology start-up developed in 2020. It has a more hybrid approach in terms of digital modules on all aspects of pain management, especially in terms of new habit formation. It is being trialled in a number of NHS pain clinics including mine.
- Pathway Through Pain: pathwaythroughpain.com (DIY)

Possibly the first desktop- and app-based 24-module programme available in the UK for both patients and organisations.
- Virtual group consults for pain (DWY to DIY)
These are becoming increasing popular in primary care and the community, and are run by GPs in their practices along with their teams, not just for pain but also for other long-term condition management. It might be a good idea to speak to your GP to see if they run such programmes for pain in your practice.

Patient advocate websites

- Living Well with Pain: livingwellpain.net
Website of patient advocate Tina Pierce.
- My Cuppa Jo: mycuppajo.com
Website of patient advocate, educator and speaker Joletta Belton.
- PainScience: painscience.com
Website of Paul Ingraham, author, publisher and former massage therapist.
- The Pain Toolkit: paintoolkit.org
Website of the original patient advocate and pain patient Pete Moore and The Pain Toolkit workbook and workshops.

Acknowledgements

This book has been an opportunity for me to stand on the shoulders of so many great giants in the pain world. It has been a difficult, sometimes impossible, yet ultimately rewarding task of distilling the best of their knowledge into something that a patient in my clinic would find useful. When this project started, I found myself in uncharted territory and it would have been impossible for me to achieve this finished product without the unwavering support and presence of many important people. I've had the good fortune to be surrounded and advised by so many people. If I have not mentioned your name or have missed someone out, then my deepest apologies. I never intended for it to be that way.

To my wonderful kids, Siddharth and Manya, for giving me purpose and meaning in what I do and who I do it for.

To my amazing parents, my sister, my brother-in-law and my in-laws for their unconditional support and love, and for being my biggest fans.

My everlasting love, admiration and gratitude to my wife Sharada, the stable rock in my life. She indulged me in my 'midlife crisis' and supported me not just in writing this book but also in my business studies at Henley and the associated tumult. For your unconditional love, constant support and encouragement and for soaking up the pressure of family life and giving me the freedom to pursue my dreams, thank you.

To Amer, for believing in me and seeing the potential of putting my knowledge and experience into a book and offering that value to other patients. A special thank you to Rajanikanth T.V., ENT surgeon, cartoonist extraordinaire and my dear friend, for making the time, despite his busy surgical practice, to make a skeleton resemble Rodin's *Thinker*.

To all the colleagues, patients and friends who have given their time and their energy to talk to me when I was writing this book. They include, in no particular order: Praveen Nandra, Ben Mynott, Rahul Seewal, Richard Harrison, Rupa Joshi, Pete Moore, Betsan Corkhill, Tina Price, Louise Trewern, Sean Jennings and Lucy Pickup. Thank you for allowing me to talk about you in this book. To Lucy, who has been a shining example of how adversity can be successfully challenged with the power of inner resilience. Special thanks to Betsan and Harriet especially who read big chunks of these chapters and gave me important feedback. I'd like to thank many of my patients and my colleagues who read the early versions of this book – it has benefited immensely from this. Thank you all. You know who you are.

To my amazing colleagues (nurses/physiotherapists/psychology/admin staff and fellow consultants) at the Royal Berkshire Hospital and the IPASS service. You have been silent witnesses and supporters in all my ideas, encouraging my vision and dreams. I cannot thank you enough. I have learnt so much about patients and their care and it has revolutionised my way of looking at pain patients and understanding them much better.

Many thanks to inspirational teachers and mentors like Joe Tatta, Arun Bhaskar, Rajesh Munglani, Ravi Kumar and Rangu Iyer for all their advice, mentorship, guidance and feedback at critical times of not just this book-writing but also in life.

Special thanks to Joe Tatta, author of *Healing Your Pain* and Director of the Integrative Pain Science Institute, for giving me permission to reproduce the pro-inflammatory and healthy diet quizzes in Chapter 6. A number of my recommendations and knowledge are due to the Functional Nutrition for Chronic Pain Course run by Joe. It is an excellent, well-compiled resource for healthcare professionals interested in nutrition for chronic pain.

Thank you to the whole team at Vermilion who believed in me and this project and supported me throughout this period of time, in particular Sam Jackson, Julia Kellaway and Marta Catalano. I benefited from a lot of support from Julia who was able to take my really long unwieldy first draft and morph it into a magical readable work.

A big thanks to Shaa Wasmund – her online course for newbie authors gave me the confidence and ability to pitch my idea to Vermilion and the rest, as they say, is history.

Lastly but never least, to all my patients who I have looked after in the last 25 years of my medical career and who have taught me in immeasurable and numerous ways all the myriad forms in which pain can present. For that I'm eternally grateful and indebted. Thanks especially to Alice Gostomski and all the members of the fibromyalgia support group in Reading.

I can only marvel at the ability of so many of my pain patients to overcome all odds and live a richer quality of life. There are many other patients who shared their stories of how they manage their pain and cope with life and resiliently became pain-free, but there simply wasn't room in this book for all those stories. Thank you for sparing the time.

Endnotes

Introduction

1   Trachsel, L. A., Cascella, M., 2020. 'Pain theory.' StatPearls Publishing. Retrieved from https://www.ncbi.nlm.nih.gov/books/NBK545194/.

2   HQIP and the British Pain Society. 'National pain audit final report 2010–2012.' Retrieved from https://www.britishpainsociety.org/static/uploads/resources/files/members_articles_npa_2012_1.pdf (accessed 30 Aug. 2020).

3   National Institute for Health and Clinical Excellence. 'Chronic pain: Assessment and Management' [in development]. Retrieved from https://www.nice.org.uk/guidance/indevelopment/gid-ng10069/consultation/html-content-2 (accessed 10 Aug. 2020).

4   Fayaz, A., Croft, P., Langford, R. M., Donaldson, L. J. and Jones, G. T., 2016. 'Prevalence of chronic pain in the UK: A systematic review and meta-analysis of population studies.' *BMJ Open*, 6(6), p. e010364.

Chapter 1

1   International Association for the Study of Pain, 2020. 'A revised definition of pain.' Retrieved from http://s3.amazonaws.com/rdcms-iasp/files/production/public/Revised%20Definition%20of%20Pain_Translations.pdf (accessed 6 Sep. 2020).

Chapter 2

1   Ofri, D., 2017. *What Patients Say, What Doctors Hear.* Beacon Press.

2   Nicholas, M. K., 2007. 'The pain self-efficacy questionnaire: Taking pain into account.' *European Journal of Pain*, 11(2), pp. 153–63.

Chapter 3

1   Live Well With Pain, 2019. 'A new film to inspire your patients.' Retrieved from https://livewellwithpain.co.uk/news/a-new-film-to-inspire-your-patients/ (accessed 29 Aug. 2020).

2   International Association for the Study of Pain, 2019. 'World Health Assembly of the WHO approves 11th version of the International Classification of Diseases (ICD-11), including new diagnostic codes for chronic pain.' Retrieved from http://s3.amazonaws.com/rdcms-iasp/files/production/public/ICD11%20Press%20Release_3June2019.pdf (accessed 29 Aug. 2020).

3   Barke, A., 2019. 'Chronic pain has arrived in the ICD-11.' International Association for the Study of Pain. Retrieved from https://www.iasp-pain.org/PublicationsNews/NewsDetail.aspx?ItemNumber=8340 (accessed 29 Aug. 2020).

4   Moseley, L., 2014. 'TEDx Adelaide Lorimer Moseley Why Things Hurt' [video]. YouTube. Retrieved from https://www.youtube.com/watch?v=gwd-wLdlHjs (accessed 6 Sep. 2020).

5   National Institute for Health and Clinical Excellence, 2020. 'Commonly used treatments for chronic pain can do more harm than good and should not be used, says NICE in draft guidance.' Retrieved from https://www.nice.org.uk/news/article/commonly-used-treatments-for-chronic-pain-can-do-more-harm-than-good-and-should-not-be-used-says-nice-in-draft-guidance (accessed 29 Aug. 2020).

6   Moore, P., 2019. 'Dr Tim Williams 10 top tips for managing pain – A guide for GP's [sic].' The Pain Toolkit. Retrieved from https://www.paintoolkit.org/news/article/dr-tim-williams-10-top-tips-for-managing-pain-a-guide-for-gps (accessed 29 Aug. 2020).

7   Faculty of Pain Medicine, 2020. 'Dose equivalents and changing opioids.' Retrieved from https://fpm.ac.uk/opioids-aware-structured-approach-opioid-prescribing/dose-equivalents-and-changing-opioids (accessed 29 Aug. 2020); Faculty of Pain Medicine, [n.d.]. 'The role of medication in pain management.' Retrieved from https://www.fpm.ac.uk/opioids-aware-understanding-pain-medicines-pain/role-medication-pain-management (accessed 29 Aug. 2020).

8   Lipton, R. B., Göbel, H., Einhäupl, K. M., Wilks, K. and Mauskop, A., 2004. '*Petasites hybridus* root (butterbur) is an effective preventive treatment for migraine.' *Neurology*, *63*(12), pp. 2240–4.

9 FNPA, [n.d.]. 'The anti-inflammatory power of cat's claw.' Retrieved from https://www.fnpa.org/the-anti-inflammatory-power-of-cats-claw/ (accessed 1 Oct. 2020).

10 Leong, D. J., Choudhury, M., Hanstein, R., Hirsh, D. M., Kim, S. J., Majeska, R. J., Schaffler, M. B., Hardin, J. A., Spray, D. C., Goldring, M. B., Cobelli, N. J. and Sun, H. B., 2014. 'Green tea polyphenol treatment is chondroprotective, anti-inflammatory and palliative in a mouse post-traumatic osteoarthritis model.' *Arthritis Research & Therapy*, 16(6), p. 508.

11 Moore, A., Derry, S., Eccleston, C. and Kalso, E., 2013. 'Expect analgesic failure; pursue analgesic success.' *BMJ*, 346(may03 1), p. f2690.

12 Government of Western Australia, Department of Health, 2016. 'Pain health.' Retrieved from https://painhealth.csse.uwa.edu.au/wp-content/uploads/2016/04/painHEALTH-NNT-and-NNH-for-pain-medications.pdf (accessed 29 Aug. 2020); Perry, D. and Allen, M., 2018. 'Topical capsaicin for neuropathic and osteoarthritis pain: Maybe not so hot?' Retrieved from https://gomainpro.ca/wp-content/uploads/tools-for-practice/1544426278_tfp225capsaicinfv.pdf (accessed 29 Aug. 2020); Teater, D., 2020. 'Evidence for efficacy of pain medications.' Retrieved from https://www.nsc.org/Portals/0/Documents/RxDrugOverdoseDocuments/Evidence-Efficacy-Pain-Medications.pdf (accessed 29 Aug. 2020); Moore, R., Derry, S., Aldington, D. and Wiffen, P., 2015. 'Single dose oral analgesics for acute postoperative pain in adults – an overview of Cochrane reviews.' Cochrane Database of Systematic Reviews (9); Bandolier, [n.d.]. 'Oxford league table of analgesics in acute pain.' Retrieved from http://www.bandolier.org.uk/booth/painpag/Acutrev/Analgesics/Leagtab.html (accessed 29 Aug. 2020); Bandolier, [n.d.]. 'Oral codeine in acute postoperative pain.' Retrieved from http://www.bandolier.org.uk/booth/painpag/Acutrev/Analgesics/AP006.html (accessed 29 Aug. 2020).

13 Moore, A., Derry, S., Eccleston, C. and Kalso, E., 2013. 'Expect analgesic failure; pursue analgesic success.' *BMJ*, 346(may03 1), p. f2690.

14 Baldini, A., Von Korff, M. and Lin, E. H., 2012. 'A review of potential adverse effects of long-term opioid therapy: A practitioner's guide.' *The Primary Care Companion for CNS Disorders*, 14(3), PCC.11m01326.

15 Cahill, C. M. and Taylor, A. M., 2017. 'Neuroinflammation – A co-occurring phenomenon linking chronic pain and opioid dependence.' *Current Opinion in Behavioral Sciences*, 13, pp. 171–7.

16 De Weerdt, S., 2019. 'Tracing the US opioid crisis to its roots.' Nature. Retrieved from https://www.nature.com/articles/d41586-019-02686-2 (accessed 29 Aug. 2020).

17 Alexander, B., Coambs, R. and Hadaway, P., 1978. 'The effect of housing and gender on morphine self-administration in rats.' *Psychopharmacology*, 58(2), pp. 175–9.

18 Robins, L., Davis, D. and Goodwin, D., 1974. 'Drug use by US army enlisted men in Vietnam: A follow-up on their return home.' *American Journal of Epidemiology*, 99(4), pp. 235–49; Robins, L., Helzer, J., Hesselbrock, M. and Wish, E., 2010. 'Vietnam veterans three years after Vietnam: How our study changed our view of heroin.' *American Journal on Addiction*s, 19(3), pp. 203–11.

19 Maté, D., 2018. *In The Realm of Hungry Ghosts*. Vermilion.

20 Hari, J., 2015. 'Everything you think you know about addiction is wrong' [video]. TED. Retrieved from https://www.ted.com/talks/johann_hari_everything_you_think_you_know_about_addiction_is_wrong?language=en (accessed 30 Aug. 2020).

21 Reproduced with permission: Webster, L. R. and Webster, R. M., 2005. 'Predicting aberrant behaviors in opioid-treated patients: Preliminary validation of the opioid risk tool.' *Pain Medicine*, 6(6), pp. 432–42.

22 Kaptchuk, T., Friedlander, E., Kelley, J., Sanchez, M., Kokkotou, E., Singer, J., Kowalczykowski, M., Miller, F., Kirsch, I. and Lembo, A., 2010. 'Placebos without deception: A randomized controlled trial in irritable bowel syndrome.' *PLoS ONE*, 5(12), p. e15591.

23 Corner, N., 2018. 'Proof positive thinking can cure our pain? Dr Michael Mosley gives 117 unwitting volunteers placebo pills to treat their chronic back problems – and almost half say it worked.' *Mail Online*. Retrieved from https://www.dailymail.co.uk/femail/article-6236423/UKs-biggest-experiment-gives-117-people-placebo-drug-nearly-HALF-cured.html (accessed 30 Aug. 2020).

24 Colloca, L., 2017. 'Nocebo effects can make you feel pain.' *Science*, 358(6359), p. 44.

Chapter 4

1 Harris, I., 2016. *Surgery, The Ultimate Placebo: A Surgeon Cuts Through The Evidence*. UNSW [first ed.].

2 Goldenberg, D., 2017. 'Osteoarthritis and central pain. Practical Pain Management. Retrieved from https://www.practicalpainmanagement.com/pain/myofascial/osteoarthritis/osteoarthritis-central-pain (accessed 30 Aug. 2020).

3 Harris, I., 2016. *Surgery, The Ultimate Placebo: A Surgeon Cuts Through The Evidence*. UNSW [first ed.].

4   Ibid.

5   Briggs, E., Battelli, D., Gordon, D., Kopf, A., Ribeiro, S., Puig, M. and Kress, H., 2015. 'Current pain education within undergraduate medical studies across Europe: Advancing the Provision of Pain Education and Learning (APPEAL) study.' *BMJ Open*, 5(8), p. e006984.

6   Ibid.

7   Firanescu, C., de Vries, J., Lodder, P., Venmans, A., Schoemaker, M., Smeet, A., Donga, E., Juttmann, J., Klazen, C., Elgersma, O., Jansen, F., Tielbeek, A., Boukrab, I., Schonenberg, K., van Rooij, W., Hirsch, J. and Lohle, P., 2018. 'Vertebroplasty versus sham procedure for painful acute osteoporotic vertebral compression fractures (VERTOS IV): Randomised sham controlled clinical trial.' *BMJ*, p. k1551.

8   Louw, A., Diener, I., Fernández-de-las-Peñas, C. and Puentedura, E., 2017. 'Sham surgery in orthopedics: A systematic review of the literature. *Pain Medicine*, p. pnw164.

9   International Association for the Study of Pain, 2017. 'Pain after surgery.' Retrieved from https://www.iasp-pain.org/GlobalYear/AfterSurgery (accessed 30 Aug. 2020); Inoue, S., Kamiya, M., Nishihara, M., Arai, Y., Ikemoto, T. and Ushida, T., 2017. 'Prevalence, characteristics, and burden of failed back surgery syndrome: The influence of various residual symptoms on patient satisfaction and quality of life as assessed by a nationwide Internet survey in Japan.' *Journal of Pain Research*, 10, pp. 811–23; Richebé, P., Capdevila, X. and Rivat, C., 2018. 'Persistent postsurgical pain.' *Anesthesiology*, 129(3), pp. 590–607; Wylde, V., Beswick, A., Bruce, J., Blom, A., Howells, N. and Gooberman-Hill, R., 2018. 'Chronic pain after total knee arthroplasty.' *EFORT Open Reviews*, 3(8), pp. 461–70.

10 Lavand'Homme, P. and Pogatzki-Zahn, E., 2017. 'Fact sheet no. 4: Chronic postsurgical pain: Definition, impact, and prevention.' International Association for the Study of Pain. Retrieved from https://s3.amazonaws.com/rdcms-iasp/files/production/public/2017GlobalYear/FactSheets/4.%20Chronic%20Postsurgical%20Pain.LavandHomme-Zahn-EE_1485789834697_3.pdf (accessed 30 Aug. 2020).

11 Macrae, W., 2001. 'Chronic pain after surgery.' *British Journal of Anaesthesia*, 87(1), pp. 88–98.

12 Lavand'Homme, P. and Pogatzki-Zahn, E., 2017. 'Fact sheet no. 4: Chronic postsurgical pain: Definition, impact, and prevention.' International Association for the Study of Pain. Retrieved from https://s3.amazonaws.com/rdcms-iasp/files/production/public/2017GlobalYear/FactSheets/4.%20Chronic%20Postsurgical%20Pain.LavandHomme-Zahn-EE_1485789834697_3.pdf (accessed 30 Aug. 2020).

13 Setchell, J., Costa, N., Ferreira, M., Makovey, J., Nielsen, M. and Hodges, P. W., 2017. 'Individuals' explanations for their persistent or recurrent low back pain: a cross-sectional survey.' *BMC Musculoskeletal Disorders*, 18(1), p. 466.

14 Prasad, V. and Cifu, A., 2015. *Ending Medical Reversal*. Johns Hopkins University Press; Harris, I., 2016. *Surgery, The Ultimate Placebo: A Surgeon Cuts Through The Evidence*. UNSW [first ed.].

15 Choosing Wisely UK, [n.d.]. 'About Choosing Wisely UK.' Retrieved from https://www.choosingwisely.co.uk/about-choosing-wisely-uk/ (accessed 30 Aug. 2020).

Chapter 5

1 Darnall, B. D., Carr, D. B. and Schatman, M. E., 2017. 'Pain psychology and the biopsychosocial model of pain treatment: Ethical imperatives and social responsibility.' *Pain Medicine*, 18(8), pp. 1413–15.

2 Fisher, J., Hassan, D. and O'Connor, N., 1995. 'Minerva.' *BMJ*, 310(6971), p. 70.

3 Dimsdale, J. and Dantzer, R., 2007. 'A biological substrate for somatoform disorders: Importance of pathophysiology. *Psychosomatic Medicine*, 69(9), pp. 850–4.

4 Ingraham, P., 2020. 'Pain is weird: A volatile, misleading sensation.' PainScience.com. Retrieved from https://www.painscience.com/articles/pain-is-weird.php (accessed 30 Aug. 2020).

5 Beecher, H., 1956. 'Relationship of significance of wound to pain experienced.' *Journal of the American Medical Association*, 161(17), p. 1609.

6 Moseley, G. and Butler, D., 2015. *The Explain Pain Handbook*. NOI Group [first ed.]; Moseley, G. and Butler, D., 2017. *Explain Pain Supercharged*. NOI Group [first ed.].

7 Shipton, E., Bate, F., Garrick, R., Steketee, C., Shipton, E. and Visser, E., 2018. 'Systematic review of pain medicine content, teaching, and assessment in medical school curricula internationally.' *Pain and Therapy*, 7(2), pp. 139–61.

8 Wall, P. and McMahon, S., 1986. 'The relationship of perceived pain to afferent nerve impulses.' *Trends in Neurosciences*, 9, pp. 254–5.

9 Doidge, N., 2015. *The Brain's Way of Healing*. Penguin US [first ed.].

10 Hargrove, T., 2016. 'Predictive coding: Why expectation matters for movement and pain.' Better Movement. Retrieved from https://www.better movement.org/blog/2016/predictive-processing (accessed 30 Aug. 2020).

11 Peters, S., 2018. *The Silent Guides*. Lagom [first ed.].

12 Felitti, V., Anda, R., Nordenberg, D., Williamson, D., Spitz, A., Edwards, V., Koss, M. and Marks, J., 1998. 'Relationship of childhood abuse and household dysfunction to many of the leading causes of death in adults.' *American Journal of Preventive Medicine*, 14(4), pp. 245–58.

13 Nicol, A. L., Sieberg, C. B., Clauw, D. J., Hassett, A. L., Moser, S. E. and Brummett, C. M., 2016. 'The association between a history of lifetime traumatic events and pain severity, physical function, and affective distress in patients with chronic pain.' *The Journal of Pain*, 17(12), pp. 1334–48.

14 Ramachandran, V., 2012. *The Tell-Tale Brain*. Windmill Books.

15 Stanton, T., Gilpin, H., Edwards, L., Moseley, G. and Newport, R., 2018. 'Illusory resizing of the painful knee is analgesic in symptomatic knee osteoarthritis.' *PeerJ*, 6, p. e5206.

16 Stanton, T., Moseley, L., Wong, A. and Kawchuk, G., 2017. 'Feeling stiffness in the back: A protective perceptual inference in chronic back pain.' *Scientific Reports*, 7(1).

17 Eisenberger, N., 2003. 'Does rejection hurt? An fMRI study of social exclusion.' *Science*, 302(5643), pp. 290–2; Taylor, J., 2016. 'Mirror neurons after a quarter century: New light, new cracks.' Science in the News. Retrieved from http://sitn.hms.harvard.edu/flash/2016/mirror-neurons-quarter-century-new-light-new-cracks/ (accessed 31 Aug. 2020).

18 Dworsky-Fried, Z., Kerr, B. and Taylor, A., 2020. 'Microbes, microglia, and pain.' *Neurobiology of Pain*, 7, p. 100045; Lurie, D., 2018. 'An integrative approach to neuroinflammation in psychiatric disorders and neuropathic pain.' *Journal of Experimental Neuroscience*, 12, p. 117906951879363.

19 Porges, S., 2009. 'The polyvagal theory: New insights into adaptive reactions of the autonomic nervous system.' *Cleveland Clinic Journal of Medicine*, 76(4 suppl 2), pp. S86–90.

20 Chen, G., Zhang, Y., Qadri, Y., Serhan, C. and Ji, R., 2018. 'Microglia in pain: Detrimental and protective roles in pathogenesis and resolution of pain.' *Neuron*, 100(6), pp. 1292–311; Kato, T. and Kanba, S., 2013. 'Are microglia minding us? Digging up the unconscious mind-brain relationship from a neuropsychoanalytic approach.' *Frontiers in Human Neuroscience*, 7; Nakazawa, D., 2020. *The Angel and the Assassin*. Ballantine Books [first ed.]; Dworsky-Fried, Z., Kerr, B. and Taylor, A., 2020. 'Microbes, microglia, and pain.' *Neurobiology of Pain*, 7, p. 100045; Fumagalli, M., Lombardi, M., Gressens, P. and Verderio, C., 2018. 'How to reprogram microglia toward beneficial functions.' *Glia*, 66(12), pp. 2531–49.

21   Chen, G., Zhang, Y., Qadri, Y., Serhan, C. and Ji, R., 2018. 'Microglia in pain: Detrimental and protective roles in pathogenesis and resolution of pain.' *Neuron*, *100*(6), pp. 1292–311.

22   Nakazawa, D., 2020. *The Angel and the Assassin*. Ballantine Books [first ed.].

23   Moseley, G. and Butler, D., 2017. *Explain Pain Supercharged*. NOI Group.

24   Bower, J. and Irwin, M., 2016. 'Mind–body therapies and control of inflammatory biology: A descriptive review.' *Brain, Behavior, and Immunity*, *51*, pp. 1–11.

25   Caudill, M., 2015. *Managing Pain Before It Manages You*. Guildford Press [fourth ed.].

Chapter 6

1   Mayer, E., 2018. *The Mind–Gut Connection: How the Hidden Conversation Within Our Bodies Impacts Our Mood, Our Choices, and Our Overall Health*. HarperCollins Publishers Inc.; Collen, A., 2015. *10% Human: How Your Body's Microbes Hold the Key to Health and Happiness*. William Collins [first ed.].

2   Collen, A., 2015. *10% Human: How Your Body's Microbes Hold the Key to Health and Happiness*. William Collins [first ed.].

3   Nijs, J., Elma, Ö., Yilmaz, S., Mullie, P., Vanderweeën, L., Clarys, P., Deliens, T., Coppieters, I., Weltens, N., Van Oudenhove, L. and Malfliet, A., 2019. 'Nutritional neurobiology and central nervous system sensitisation: Missing link in a comprehensive treatment for chronic pain?' *British Journal of Anaesthesia*, *123*(5), pp. 539–43.

4   Dworsky-Fried, Z., Kerr, B. and Taylor, A., 2020. 'Microbes, microglia, and pain.' *Neurobiology of Pain*, 7, p. 100045.

5   Enders, G., 2015. *Gut*. Scribe.

6   Yano, J., Yu, K., Donaldson, G., Shastri, G., Ann, P., Ma, L., Nagler, C., Ismagilov, R., Mazmanian, S. and Hsiao, E., 2015. 'Indigenous bacteria from the gut microbiota regulate host serotonin biosynthesis.' *Cell*, *161*(2), pp.264–76.

7   Guo, R., Chen, L., Xing, C. and Liu, T., 2019. 'Pain regulation by gut microbiota: Molecular mechanisms and therapeutic potential.' *British Journal of Anaesthesia*, *123*(5), pp. 637–54.

8   Luczynski, P., Tramullas, M., Viola, M., Shanahan, F., Clarke, G., O'Mahony, S., Dinan, T. G. and Cryan, J. F., 2017. 'Microbiota regulates visceral pain in the mouse.' *eLife*, 6, p. e25887.

9   Boer, C., Radjabzadeh, D., Uitterlinden, A., Kraaij, R. and van Meurs, J., 2017. 'The role of the gut microbiome in osteoarthritis and joint pain.' *Osteoarthritis and Cartilage, 25*, p. S10.

10 Mayer, E., 2018. *The Mind–Gut Connection: How the Hidden Conversation Within Our Bodies Impacts Our Mood, Our Choices, and Our Overall Health.* HarperCollins Publishers Inc.

11 Adapted from Tatta, J., 2020. '*How healthy is your diet?* Integrative Pain Science Institute.

12 Davies, A., Cretella, A., Rut, M., Franck, V. and Mackenzie, S., 2019. 'Solo dining is bad for our mental health – and for the planet.' Quartz. Retrieved from https://qz.com/1738347/eating-alone-is-bad-for-our-mental-health-and-the-planet/ (accessed 7 Oct. 2020).

13 Cunningham, S. A., Vaquera, E., Maturo, C. C. and Narayan, K. M., 2012. 'Is there evidence that friends influence body weight? A systematic review of empirical research.' *Social Science & Medicine, 75*(7), pp. 1175–83.

14 McVinnie, D., 2013. 'Obesity and pain.' *British Journal of Pain, 7*(4), pp. 163–70.

15 Stone, A. and Broderick, J., 2012. 'Obesity and pain are associated in the United States.' *Obesity, 20*(7), pp. 1491–5.

16 Leboeuf-Yde, C., Kyvik, K. and Bruun, N., 1999. 'Low back pain and lifestyle. Part II – Obesity.' *Spine, 24*(8), pp.779–84.

17 Hagen, K., Linde, M., Heuch, I., Stovner, L. and Zwart, J., 2011. 'Increasing prevalence of chronic musculoskeletal complaints. A large 11-year follow-up in the general population (HUNT 2 and 3).' *Pain Medicine, 12*(11), pp. 1657–66.

18 Tatta, J., 2020. '*How healthy is your diet?* Integrative Pain Science Institute.

19 NHS, 2020. 'Sugar: The facts.' Retrieved from https://www.nhs.uk/live-well/eat-well/how-does-sugar-in-our-diet-affect-our-health/ (accessed 2 Sep. 2020).

20 Public Health Collaboration, 2020. 'Sugar equivalent infographics courtesy of Dr David Unwin.' Retrieved from https://phcuk.org/sugar/ (accessed 2 Sep. 2020).

21 Soliman, G., 2018. 'Dietary Cholesterol and the lack of evidence in cardiovascular disease.' *Nutrients, 10*(6), p. 780.

22 ChooseMyPlate, [n.d.]. 'Saturated fat.' Retrieved from https://www.heartuk.org.uk/low-cholesterol-foods/saturated-fat (accessed 5 Jan. 2021).

23 Pesticide Action Network UK, 2019. 'Pesticides in our food.' Retrieved from https://www.pan-uk.org/site/wp-content/uploads/Pesticides-in-our-food-multiple-residues-June-2019-1.pdf (accessed 1 Sep. 2020).

24 Pesticide Action Network UK, 2019. 'The dirty dozen and clean fifteen.' Retrieved from https://www.pan-uk.org/dirty-dozen-and-clean-fifteen/ (accessed 1 Sep. 2020).

25 Brain, K., Burrows, T., Rollo, M., Chai, L., Clarke, E., Hayes, C., Hodson, F. and Collins, C., 2018. 'A systematic review and meta-analysis of nutrition interventions for chronic noncancer pain.' *Journal of Human Nutrition and Dietetics*, 32(2), pp. 198–225.

26 Tick, H., 2013. *Holistic Pain Relief*. New World Library.

27 Tatta, J., 2019. 'Functional nutrition for chronic pain' [online course].

28 Thurm, T., Ablin, J. N., Buskila, D. and Maharshak, N., 2017. 'Fecal microbiota transplantation for fibromyalgia: A case report and review of the literature.' *Open Journal of Gastroenterology*, 7(4), pp. 131–9.

29 Panda, S., 2017. 'Health lies in healthy circadian habits' [transcript]. TED. Retrieved from https://www.ted.com/talks/satchin_panda_health_lies_in_healthy_circadian_habits/transcript?language=en (accessed 2 Sep. 2020).

30 Longo, V. and Panda, S., 2016. 'Fasting, circadian rhythms, and time-restricted feeding in healthy lifespan.' *Cell Metabolism*, 23(6), pp. 1048–59.

Chapter 7

1 Adapted from Kelly, J. and Shull, J., 2019. *Foundations of Lifestyle Medicine: The Lifestyle Medicine Board Review Manual*. American College of Lifestyle Medicine, p. 276.

2 Walker, M., 2018. *Why We Sleep*. Penguin [first ed.].

3 Kwekkeboom, K., Cherwin, C., Lee, J. and Wanta, B., 2010. 'Mind-body treatments for the pain-fatigue-sleep disturbance symptom cluster in persons with cancer.' *Journal of Pain and Symptom Management*, 39(1), pp. 126–38.

4 Keilani, M., Crevenna, R. and Dorner, T., 2017. 'Sleep quality in subjects suffering from chronic pain.' *Wiener klinische Wochenschrift*, 130(1–2), pp. 31–6.

5 Finan, P., Goodin, B. and Smith, M., 2013. 'The association of sleep and pain: An update and a path forward.' *The Journal of Pain*, 14(12), pp. 1539–52.

6 Finan, P., Quartana, P. and Smith, M., 2015. 'The effects of sleep continuity disruption on positive mood and sleep architecture in healthy adults.' *Sleep*, 38(11), pp. 1735–42.

7   Finan, P., Goodin, B. and Smith, M., 2013. 'The association of sleep and pain: An update and a path forward.' *The Journal of Pain*, *14*(12), pp. 1539–52; Keilani, M., Crevenna, R. and Dorner, T., 2017. 'Sleep quality in subjects suffering from chronic pain.' *Wiener klinische Wochenschrift*, *130*(1–2), pp. 31–6.

8   Keilani, M., Crevenna, R. and Dorner, T., 2017. 'Sleep quality in subjects suffering from chronic pain.' *Wiener klinische Wochenschrift*, *130*(1–2), pp. 31–6.

9   Jank, R., Gallee, A., Boeckle, M., Fiegl, S. and Pieh, C., 2017. 'Chronic pain and sleep disorders in primary care.' *Pain Research and Treatment*, pp. 1–9.

10 Finan, P., Goodin, B. and Smith, M., 2013. 'The association of sleep and pain: An update and a path forward.' *The Journal of Pain*, *14*(12), pp. 1539–52.

11 Carley, D. and Farabi, S., 2016. 'Physiology of sleep.' *Diabetes Spectrum*, *29*(1), pp. 5–9.

12 Olson, K., 2015. 'Pain and sleep: Understanding the interrelationship.' Practical Pain Management. Retrieved from https://www.practical painmanagement.com/pain/other/co-morbidities/pain-sleep-understanding-interrelationship (accessed 1 Sep. 2020).

13 He, Y., Jones, C., Fujiki, N., Xu, Y., Guo, B., Holder, J., Rossner, M., Nishino, S. and Fu, Y., 2009. 'The transcriptional repressor DEC2 regulates sleep length in mammals.' *Science*, *325*(5942), pp. 866–70.

14 Walker, M., 2018. *Why We Sleep*. Penguin [first ed.]; Jank, R., Gallee, A., Boeckle, M., Fiegl, S. and Pieh, C., 2017. 'Chronic pain and sleep disorders in primary care.' *Pain Research and Treatment*, pp. 1–9.

15 Buscemi, N., Vandermeer, B., Friesen, C., Bialy, L., Tubman, M., Ospina, M., Klassen, T. P. and Witmans, M., 2007. 'The efficacy and safety of drug treatments for chronic insomnia in adults: A meta-analysis of RCTs.' *Journal of General Internal Medicine*, *22*(9), pp. 1335–50.

16 Walker, M., 2018. *Why We Sleep*. Penguin [first ed.].

17 Ibid.

18 Kwekkeboom, K., Cherwin, C., Lee, J. and Wanta, B., 2010. 'Mind-body treatments for the pain-fatigue-sleep disturbance symptom cluster in persons with cancer.' *Journal of Pain and Symptom Management*, *39*(1), pp. 126–38.

19 Qaseem, A., Kansagara, D., Forciea, M., Cooke, M. and Denberg, T., 2016. 'Management of chronic insomnia disorder in adults: A clinical practice guideline from the American College of Physicians.' *Annals of Internal Medicine*, *165*(2), p. 125.

20 Amutio, A., Franco, C., Sánchez-Sánchez, L. C., Pérez-Fuentes, M., Gázquez-Linares, J. J., Van Gordon, W. and Molero-Jurado, M., 2018. 'Effects of mindfulness training on sleep problems in patients with fibromyalgia.' *Frontiers in Psychology*, 9, p. 1365.

21 Ablin, J. N., Häuser, W. and Buskila, D., 2013. 'Spa treatment (balneotherapy) for fibromyalgia – A qualitative-narrative review and a historical perspective.' *Evidence-based Complementary and Alternative Medicine*, 2013, p. 638050.

22 Suni, E., 2020. 'Sleep hygiene.' SleepFoundation.org. Retrieved from https://www.sleepfoundation.org/articles/sleep-hygiene (accessed 2 Sep. 2020).

Chapter 8

1 Endrighi, R., Steptoe, A. and Hamer, M., 2016. 'The effect of experimentally induced sedentariness on mood and psychobiological responses to mental stress.' *British Journal of Psychiatry*, 208(3), pp. 245–51.

2 Geneen, L., Moore, R., Clarke, C., Martin, D., Colvin, L. and Smith, B., 2017. 'Physical activity and exercise for chronic pain in adults: An overview of Cochrane Reviews.' *Cochrane Database of Systematic Review* (4).

3 Lee, I., Shiroma, E., Lobelo, F., Puska, P., Blair, S. and Katzmarzyk, P., 2012. 'Effect of physical inactivity on major non-communicable diseases worldwide: An analysis of burden of disease and life expectancy.' *The Lancet*, 380(9838), pp. 219–29.

4 World Health Organization, 2020. 'Physical inactivity: A global public health problem.' Retrieved from https://www.who.int/ncds/prevention/physical-activity/inactivity-global-health-problem/en/#:~:text=Globally%2C%2023%25%20of%20adults%20and,80%25%20in%20some%20adult%20subpopulations. (accessed 5 Jan. 2021).

5 Moving Medicine, [n.d.]. 'Why moving matters.' Retrieved from https://movingmedicine.ac.uk/why-movement-matters/why-moving-matters-2/ (accessed 5 Jan. 2021).

6 Holmes, B., 2020. 'Movement as medicine.' The Week. Retrieved from https://theweek.com/articles/888296/movement-medicine (accessed 2 Sep. 2020).

7 Leal, L., Lopes, M. and Batista, M., 2018. 'Physical exercise-induced myokines and muscle-adipose tissue crosstalk: A review of current knowledge and the implications for health and metabolic diseases.' *Frontiers in Physiology*, 9.

8   Kurth, F., Cherbuin, N. and Luders, E., 2017. 'Promising links between meditation and reduced (brain) aging: An attempt to bridge some gaps between the alleged fountain of youth and the youth of the field.' *Frontiers in Psychology*, 8.

9   Garatachea, N., Pareja-Galeano, H., Sanchis-Gomar, F., Santos-Lozano, A., Fiuza-Luces, C., Morán, M., Emanuele, E., Joyner, M. J. and Lucia, A., 2015. 'Exercise attenuates the major hallmarks of aging.' *Rejuvenation Research*, 18(1), pp. 57–89.

10 Back to Motion, [n.d.]. 'Movement is medicine.' Retrieved from https://backtomotion.net/movement-is-medicine/ (accessed 2 Sep. 2020).

11 Suzuki, W., 2017. 'The brain-changing benefits of exercise.' TED. Retrieved from https://www.ted.com/talks/wendy_suzuki_the_brain_changing_benefits_of_exercise?language=en (accessed 2 Sep. 2020).

12 McGonigal, K., 2019. *The Joy of Movement*. Avery [first ed.].

13 Netz, Y., 2017. 'Is the comparison between exercise and pharmacologic treatment of depression in the clinical practice guideline of the American College of Physicians evidence-based?' *Frontiers in Pharmacology*, 8(257).

14 NHS, 2019. 'Exercise.' Retrieved from https://www.nhs.uk/live-well/exercise/ (accessed 2 Sep. 2020).

15 Richards, W., [n.d.]. 'Fearless fitness: An exercise guide for people with chronic pain.' Curable. Retrieved from https://www.curablehealth.com/blog/exercise-for-chronic-pain (accessed 2 Sep. 2020).

16 Dweck, C., 2012. *Mindset*. Robinson.

17 Integrative Pain Science Institute, [n.d.]. 'How and why to exercise with chronic pain.' Retrieved from https://www.integrativepainscienceinstitute.com/exercise-chronic-pain/ (accessed 2 Sep. 2020).

18 O'Sullivan, P., Caneiro, J., O'Keeffe, M., Smith, A., Dankaerts, W., Fersum, K. and O'Sullivan, K., 2018. 'Cognitive functional therapy: An integrated behavioral approach for the targeted management of disabling low back pain.' *Physical Therapy*, 98(5), pp. 408–23.

19 NHS, 2019. 'Exercise.' Retrieved from https://www.nhs.uk/live-well/exercise/ (accessed 2 Sep. 2020).

20 McGonigal, K., 2019. *The Joy of Movement*. Avery [first ed.].

21 Thompson, B., 2020. 'Is exercise the new snake oil? Or just a dirty word?' [blog]. HealthSkills. Retrieved from https://healthskills.wordpress.com/2020/08/10/is-exercise-the-new-snake-oil-or-just-a-dirty-word/ (accessed 2 Sep. 2020).

Chapter 9

1   Garland, E., Brintz, C., Hanley, A., Roseen, E., Atchley, R., Gaylord, S., Faurot, K., Yaffe, J., Fiander, M. and Keefe, F., 2020. 'Mind-body therapies for opioid-treated pain.' *JAMA Internal Medicine*, 180(1), p. 91.

2   Eccleston, C., Morley, S. and Williams, A., 2013. 'Psychological approaches to chronic pain management: Evidence and challenges.' *British Journal of Anaesthesia*, 111(1), pp. 59–63.

3   Williams, A., Fisher, E., Hearn, L. and Eccleston, C., 2020. 'Psychological therapies for the management of chronic pain (excluding headache) in adults.' *Cochrane Database of Systematic Reviews* (2).

4   Louw, A., Zimney, K., Puentedura, E. and Diener, I., 2016. 'The efficacy of pain neuroscience education on musculoskeletal pain: A systematic review of the literature.' *Physiotherapy Theory and Practice*, 32(5), pp. 332–55.

5   Orr, A., 2019. *Taming Chronic Pain*. Mango Publishing.

6   Patil, S., Sen, S., Bral, M., Reddy, S., Bradley, K., Cornett, E., Fox, C. and Kaye, A., 2016. 'The role of acupuncture in pain management.' *Current Pain and Headache Reports*, 20(4).

7   Napadow, V., Kettner, N., Liu, J., Li, M., Kwong, K., Vangel, M., Makris, N., Audette, J. and Hui, K., 2007. 'Hypothalamus and amygdala response to acupuncture stimuli in carpal tunnel syndrome.' *Pain*, 130(3), pp. 254–66.

8   National Center for Complementary and Integrative Health, 2020. 'Yoga for health: What the science says.' Retrieved from https://www.nccih.nih.gov/health/providers/digest/yoga-for-health-science (accessed 5 Sep. 2020).

9   Frank, D. L., Khorshid, L., Kiffer, J. F., Moravec, C. S. and McKee, M. G., 2010. 'Biofeedback in medicine: Who, when, why and how?' *Mental Health in Family Medicine*, 7(2), pp. 85–91.

10 Sielski, R., Rief, W. and Glombiewski, J.A., 2017. 'Efficacy of biofeedback in chronic back pain: A meta-analysis. '*International Journal of Behavioral Medicine*, 24(1), pp. 25–41.

11 Elkins, G., Jensen, M. P. and Patterson, D. R., 2007. 'Hypnotherapy for the management of chronic pain.' *The International Journal of Clinical and Experimental Hypnosis*, 55(3), 275–87.

12 Tick, H., 2013. *Holistic Pain Relief*. New World Library.

13 Ibid.

14 Kochenderfer, R., 2019. 'Expressive writing: A tool for transformation, with Dr. James Pennebaker, Ph.D.' Journaling.com. Retrieved from

https://www.journaling.com/articles/expressive-writing-a-tool-for-transformation-with-dr-james-pennebaker-ph-d/ (accessed 4 Sep. 2020).

15 Christo, P., 2017. *Aches and Gains*. Bull Publishing.

16 Ibid.

17 Ibid.

18 Ibid.

19 Kamioka, H., Okada, S., Tsutani, K., Park, H., Okuizumi, H., Handa, S., Oshio, T., Park, S., Kitayuguchi, J., Abe, T., Honda, T. and Mutoh, Y., 2014. 'Effectiveness of animal-assisted therapy: A systematic review of randomized controlled trials.' *Complementary Therapies in Medicine*, 22(2), pp. 371–90.

20 Ezzo, J., 2007. 'What can be learned from Cochrane Systematic Reviews of massage that can guide future research?' *The Journal of Alternative and Complementary Medicine*, 13(2), pp. 291–6.

21 Furlan, A., Giraldo, M., Baskwill, A., Irvin, E. and Imamura, M., 2015. 'Massage for low-back pain.' *Cochrane Database of Systematic Reviews* (9).

22 Sharma, V., Manjunath, N., Nagendra, H. and Ertsey, C., 2018. 'Combination of Ayurveda and Yoga therapy reduces pain intensity and improves quality of life in patients with migraine headache.' *Complementary Therapies in Clinical Practice*, 32, pp. 85–91.

23 Mathie, R. T., Ramparsad, N., Legg, L. A., Clausen, J., Moss, S., Davidson, J. R., Messow, C. M. and McConnachie, A., 2017. 'Randomised, double-blind, placebo-controlled trials of non-individualised homeopathic treatment: systematic review and meta-analysis.' *Systematic Reviews*, 6(1), p. 63.

24 Lee, C., Crawford, C. and Hickey, A., 2014. 'Mind–body therapies for the self-management of chronic pain symptoms.' *Pain Medicine*, 15(S1), pp. S21–39.

Chapter 10

1 Clear, J., 2019. *Atomic Habits*. Random House Business; Freedom Pact, 2020. '#90: Dr Andrew Huberman – Stanford neuroscientist on the rules of long-lasting adaptive brain change' [podcast]. Retrieved from https://soundcloud.com/freedompactpodcast/90-dr-andrew-huberman-stanford-neuroscientist-on-the-rules-of-long-lasting-adaptive-brain-change (accessed 5 Sep. 2020).

2 Ibid.

3 Garratt, J., 2019. 'How to build your own neural route 66.' BetterHumans. Retrieved from https://medium.com/better-humans/how-to-build-your-own-neural-route-66-6aec3f439ebd (accessed 5 Sep. 2020).

4   Fogg, B., 2019. *Tiny Habits*. Virgin.
5   Andreatta, B., 2019. *Wired To Grow*. 7th Mind Publishing [second ed.].
6   Chatterjee, R., 2018. *The 4 Pillar Plan*. Penguin Life.

Chapter 11

1   Gauntlett-Gilbert, J. and Brook, P., 2018. 'Living well with chronic pain: The role of pain-management programmes.' *BJA Education*, *18*(1), pp. 3–7.
2   Harman, K., MacRae, M., Vallis, M. and Bassett, R., 2014. 'Working with people to make changes: A behavioural change approach used in chronic low back pain rehabilitation.' *Physiotherapy Canada*, *66*(1), pp. 82–90.
3   Prochaska, J. O. and DiClemente, C. C., 1983. 'Stages and processes of self-change of smoking: Toward an integrative model of change.' *Journal of Consulting and Clinical Psychology*, *51*(3), pp. 390–5.

Chapter 12

1   Zou, S. and Kumar, U., 2018. 'Cannabinoid receptors and the endocannabinoid system: Signaling and function in the central nervous system.' *International Journal of Molecular Sciences*, *19*(3), p. 833.
2   Fumagalli, M., Lombardi, M., Gressens, P. and Verderio, C., 2018. 'How to reprogram microglia toward beneficial functions.' *Glia*, *66*(12), pp. 2531–49.
3   Lurie, D., 2018. 'An integrative approach to neuroinflammation in psychiatric disorders and neuropathic pain.' *Journal of Experimental Neuroscience*, *12*, p. 117906951879363.
4   Ramaswamy Reddy, S. H., Reddy, R., Babu, N. C. and Ashok, G. N., 2018. 'Stem-cell therapy and platelet-rich plasma in regenerative medicines: A review on pros and cons of the technologies.' *Journal of Oral and Maxillofacial Pathology*, *22*(3), pp. 367–74.
5   Huh, Y., Ji, R. and Chen, G., 2017. 'Neuroinflammation, bone marrow stem cells, and chronic pain.' *Frontiers in Immunology*, *8*.
6   Goudra, B., Shah, D., Balu, G., Gouda, G., Balu, A., Borle, A. and Singh, P., 2017. 'Repetitive transcranial magnetic stimulation in chronic pain: A meta-analysis.' *Anesthesia: Essays and Researches*, *11*(3), p. 751.
7   Ahmadpour, N., Randall, H., Choksi, H., Gao, A., Vaughan, C. and Poronnik, P., 2019. 'Virtual reality interventions for acute and chronic

pain management.' *The International Journal of Biochemistry & Cell Biology*, *114*, p. 105568.

8   Descalzi, G., Ikegami, D., Ushijima, T., Nestler, E. J., Zachariou, V. and Narita, M., 2015. 'Epigenetic mechanisms of chronic pain.' *Trends in Neurosciences*, *38*(4), pp. 237–46.

9   Wikipedia, 2020. 'Salutogenesis.' Retrieved from https://en.wikipedia.org/wiki/Salutogenesis#:~:text=Salutogenesis%20is%20a%20medical%20approach,health%2C%20stress%2C%20and%20coping (accessed 6 Sep. 2020).

10 Jonas, W., 2018. *How Healing Works*. Scribe.

11 Maskell, J., 2020. *The Community Cure*. Lioncrest Publishing.

12 Tello, M., 2019. 'Trauma-informed care: What it is, and why it's important' [blog]. Harvard Health Publishing. Retrieved from https://www.health.harvard.edu/blog/trauma-informed-care-what-it-is-and-why-its-important-2018101613562 (accessed 6 Sep. 2020).

13 Kemp, H. I., Corner, E. and Colvin, L. A., 2020. 'Chronic pain after COVID-19: Implications for rehabilitation.' *British Journal of Anaesthesia*, *125*(4), pp. 436–40.

Appendix

THE BODY MAP

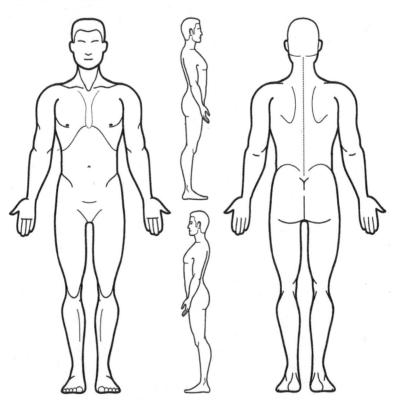

Index

Page references in *italics* indicate images.